Fit Over 40
For Dummies®

*eat
...eet*

D0775033

What Exercise Can Do for You in Your ...ge Years

- ✔ **Give you energy.** A good workout releases enzymes that make you feel great.
- ✔ **Prevent muscle deterioration.** Muscles shrink by 1 percent a year unless you embark on a consistent fitness program.
- ✔ **Make your skin look better.** Exercise increases blood flow to the skin, giving you a healthy glow.
- ✔ **Help prevent osteoporosis.** Exercise increases bone mass, which helps post-menopausal women suffering from osteoporosis.
- ✔ **Help prevent high blood pressure.** A healthy heart pumps stronger, which keeps arteries expanded.
- ✔ **Make you fitter than young couch potatoes.** Studies show that middle-aged people have lower resting heart rates than inactive people in their 20s.

You Should Consider Buying Exercise Equipment for Your Home If . . .

- ✔ You find a piece of equipment (treadmill, stair stepper, stationary bike, or elliptical machine) that you enjoy working out on.
- ✔ Your work schedule doesn't allow you time to exercise at a health club during the day.
- ✔ You don't want to be locked into a fitness club contract.
- ✔ You have a spare bedroom or den for your exercise equipment.
- ✔ You're overly self-conscious about showing your not-ready-for-prime-time legs to the world.

There Are No Good Excuses for Not Exercising

Excuse: I'm too fat.

Counterpoint: You'll weigh less if you start exercising regularly.

Excuse: I'm too tired.

Counterpoint: You won't be after you're finished exercising.

Excuse: Walking hurts my knees.

Counterpoint: Then ride a recumbent bike or swim.

Excuse: I don't have the right shoes.

Counterpoint: Sneakers are inexpensive. Buy new ones.

Excuse: I'm out of shape.

Counterpoint: So? A thousand-mile journey begins with a single step.

For Dummies™: Bestselling Book Series for Beginners

Fit Over 40 For Dummies®

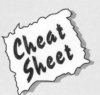

Cheat Sheet

The Fitness-Club-Tour Checklist

Ask yourself or your guide the following questions when you tour a health club or other fitness facility:

✔ **How do you like the facility as a whole?**

- **Location:** Is the club located within a 10-minute drive?

- **Age and equipment:** Does the gym have a good selection of the latest machines? Are locker space and security adequate?

- **White glove test:** Are machines dirty? Is the carpet new? Are showers clean?

- **Parking:** Is free, convenient parking available close to the front door?

- **Swimming pool:** Is the pool big enough to handle the traffic? Do they have some lanes open for swimmers during water aerobics classes?

- **Atmosphere:** Do you feel comfortable with the mix of people? How old are most of the patrons?

✔ **What's inside?**

- **Machinery:** What strength-training machines are available? Are there time constraints on how long you can stay on a particular machine?

- **Crowding:** Is the club jammed during prime workout times — 5–7 p.m.? Would it be worth the money to join a more expensive club with fewer members?

- **Classes:** Can you take different types of aerobics classes? What about classes on nutrition and weight loss? Are class schedules compatible with your work schedule?

✔ **Who's available to help?**

- **Staffing:** Does the club have several staff members around, or does one person handle the front desk, answer the phone, and sell products?

- **Fitness testing:** Can the club provide a state-of-the-art physical assessment?

- **Personal trainers:** Are personal trainers available for consultation and planning? What are their credentials?

✔ **How much will it cost?**

- **Dues:** What is the annual membership fee? Can you pay monthly or quarterly? Must you pay an initiation fee?

- **Extra fees:** Does the club charge extra to use towels? What about health or fitness classes? Does it cost more to play racquetball?

- **Guest fees:** If you want to bring a friend, what is the charge?

For Dummies™: Bestselling Book Series for Beginners

Praise for Fit Over 40 For Dummies

"This book is a must read for anyone interested in beginning or continuing an exercise program. Betsy Nagelsen McCormack has experience in all areas of training, and has put together the definitive information on this subject."

> — Richard Steadman, M.D., Steadman Hawkins Clinic

"Betsy Nagelsen McCormack is one of the fittest people I know. When I am in my forties, I will be glad I have this book."

> — Monica Seles, professional tennis player

"Few players on the women's professional tennis tour were fitter than Betsy, and I'm pleased that she has decided to share her fitness knowledge in *Fit Over 40 For Dummies.*"

> — Mary Joe Fernandez, recently retired WTA player and ESPN tennis analyst

"What a great book! Betsy gives great incentive with practical and fun tips and suggestions to get on an exercise program that not only works for anyone, but will change their life."

> — Michelle Akers, Olympic gold medallist, world champion soccer player, founder of Soccer Outreach International

"Bette Davis said, 'Old age ain't no place for sissies.' *Fit Over 40 For Dummies* says middle age is no place for excuses and helps you get off your duff and on the road to health and well-being. It's good advice and a fun read."

> — Mary Carillo, 1977 French Open mixed doubles champion, Emmy-nominated NBC commentator

"As a lifelong athlete and exercise nut, I think *Fit Over 40 For Dummies* cuts to the chase. No one can make the right choices for us. We have to be in control of our own bodies. And, if we do it right, we should have longer and healthier lives. May we all cheer Betsy when she's 100 years old as she finishes off yet another opponent on the tennis court."

> — Paula Zahn, host of *The Edge with Paula Zahn* on the FOX News Channel, former host of *The CBS News Saturday Edition* and co-host of *The CBS Morning Show*

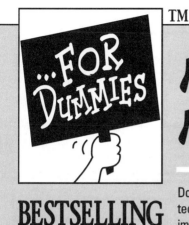
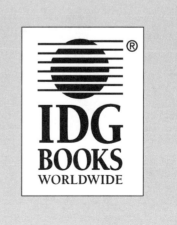

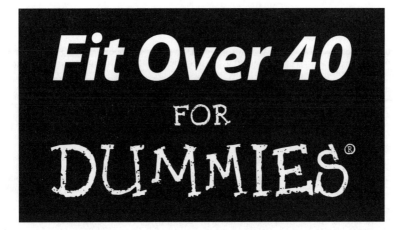

Fit Over 40 FOR DUMMIES®

by Betsy Nagelsen McCormack

with Mike Yorkey

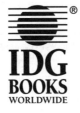

IDG
BOOKS
WORLDWIDE

IDG Books Worldwide, Inc.
An International Data Group Company

Foster City, CA ◆ Chicago, IL ◆ Indianapolis, IN ◆ New York, NY

Fit Over 40 For Dummies®

Published by
IDG Books Worldwide, Inc.
An International Data Group Company
919 E. Hillsdale Blvd.
Suite 400
Foster City, CA 94404
www.idgbooks.com (IDG Books Worldwide Web Site)
www.dummies.com (Dummies Press Web Site)

Library of Congress Control Number: 00-107694

ISBN: 0-7645-5305-4

Printed in the United States of America

10 9 8 7 6 5 4 3 2 1

1B/TR/RQ/QQ/IN

Distributed in the United States by IDG Books Worldwide, Inc.

Distributed by CDG Books Canada Inc. for Canada; by Transworld Publishers Limited in the United Kingdom; by IDG Norge Books for Norway; by IDG Sweden Books for Sweden; by IDG Books Australia Publishing Corporation Pty. Ltd. for Australia and New Zealand; by TransQuest Publishers Pte Ltd. for Singapore, Malaysia, Thailand, Indonesia, and Hong Kong; by Gotop Information Inc. for Taiwan; by ICG Muse, Inc. for Japan; by Intersoft for South Africa; by Eyrolles for France; by International Thomson Publishing for Germany, Austria and Switzerland; by Distribuidora Cuspide for Argentina; by LR International for Brazil; by Galileo Libros for Chile; by Ediciones ZETA S.C.R. Ltda. for Peru; by WS Computer Publishing Corporation, Inc., for the Philippines; by Contemporanea de Ediciones for Venezuela; by Express Computer Distributors for the Caribbean and West Indies; by Micronesia Media Distributor, Inc. for Micronesia; by Chips Computadoras S.A. de C.V. for Mexico; by Editorial Norma de Panama S.A. for Panama; by American Bookshops for Finland.

For general information on IDG Books Worldwide's books in the U.S., please call our Consumer Customer Service department at 800-762-2974. For reseller information, including discounts and premium sales, please call our Reseller Customer Service department at 800-434-3422.

For information on where to purchase IDG Books Worldwide's books outside the U.S., please contact our International Sales department at 317-572-3993 or fax 317-572-4002.

For consumer information on foreign language translations, please contact our Customer Service department at 1-800-434-3422, fax 317-572-4002, or e-mail rights@idgbooks.com.

For information on licensing foreign or domestic rights, please phone +1-650-653-7098.

For sales inquiries and special prices for bulk quantities, please contact our Order Services department at 800-434-4322 or write to the address above.

For information on using IDG Books Worldwide's books in the classroom or for ordering examination copies, please contact our Educational Sales department at 800-434-2086 or fax 317-572-4005.

For press review copies, author interviews, or other publicity information, please contact our Public Relations department at 650-653-7000 or fax 650-653-7500.

For authorization to photocopy items for corporate, personal, or educational use, please contact Copyright Clearance Center, 222 Rosewood Drive, Danvers, MA 01923, or fax 978-750-4470.

About the Authors

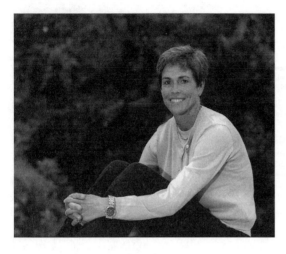

Betsy Nagelsen McCormack: Before retiring in 1996 after 23 years in professional tennis, Betsy Nagelsen McCormack earned 35 victories in singles and doubles tournaments around the world. Known by her maiden name, Betsy Nagelsen, she scored victories over Chris Evert, Martina Navratilova, Pam Shriver, and Arantxa Sanchez-Vicario, and in 1978 she lost in the finals of a Grand Slam singles event — the Australian Open. She captured two Australian Open doubles titles, but lost in the Ladies Doubles final at Wimbledon in 1987. She was once ranked as high as No. 17 in the world in singles and was a Top Ten doubles player.

During the 1990s, Betsy began a second career as a commentator for women's tennis tournaments televised by ABC Sports, ESPN, and Australia's Channel 9, and today she continues to do a wide variety of sports and health-related television work. She is a tireless volunteer for charitable organizations and devotes much of her free time to the House of Hope, a faith-based home for troubled teens in Orlando, Florida.

Betsy married Mark McCormack, founder of International Management Group (IMG), in 1986, and they are the proud parents of Maggie, a preschooler. The family resides in Windermere, Florida.

Mike Yorkey: He is the author, co-author, or general editor of more than 20 books. In addition, his magazine articles have been published in the *Los Angeles Times* travel section, *Skiing, Tennis Week, World Tennis, City Sports,* and *Racquet.*

Mike and his wife, Nicole, are the parents of two teenage children, Andrea and Patrick, and they live in Encinitas, California.

Dedication

From Betsy:

To my daughter, Maggie. May she be blessed with health, happiness, and fitness and always enjoy a good workout.

ABOUT IDG BOOKS WORLDWIDE

Welcome to the world of IDG Books Worldwide.

IDG Books Worldwide, Inc., is a subsidiary of International Data Group, the world's largest publisher of computer-related information and the leading global provider of information services on information technology. IDG was founded more than 30 years ago by Patrick J. McGovern and now employs more than 9,000 people worldwide. IDG publishes more than 290 computer publications in over 75 countries. More than 90 million people read one or more IDG publications each month.

Launched in 1990, IDG Books Worldwide is today the #1 publisher of best-selling computer books in the United States. We are proud to have received eight awards from the Computer Press Association in recognition of editorial excellence and three from Computer Currents' First Annual Readers' Choice Awards. Our best-selling ...For Dummies® series has more than 50 million copies in print with translations in 31 languages. IDG Books Worldwide, through a joint venture with IDG's Hi-Tech Beijing, became the first U.S. publisher to publish a computer book in the People's Republic of China. In record time, IDG Books Worldwide has become the first choice for millions of readers around the world who want to learn how to better manage their businesses.

Our mission is simple: Every one of our books is designed to bring extra value and skill-building instructions to the reader. Our books are written by experts who understand and care about our readers. The knowledge base of our editorial staff comes from years of experience in publishing, education, and journalism — experience we use to produce books to carry us into the new millennium. In short, we care about books, so we attract the best people. We devote special attention to details such as audience, interior design, use of icons, and illustrations. And because we use an efficient process of authoring, editing, and desktop publishing our books electronically, we can spend more time ensuring superior content and less time on the technicalities of making books.

You can count on our commitment to deliver high-quality books at competitive prices on topics you want to read about. At IDG Books Worldwide, we continue in the IDG tradition of delivering quality for more than 30 years. You'll find no better book on a subject than one from IDG Books Worldwide.

John Kilcullen
Chairman and CEO
IDG Books Worldwide, Inc.

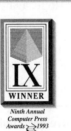

Eighth Annual
Computer Press
Awards ≥1992

Ninth Annual
Computer Press
Awards ≥1993

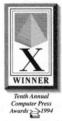

Tenth Annual
Computer Press
Awards ≥1994

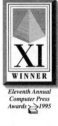

Eleventh Annual
Computer Press
Awards ≥1995

IDG is the world's leading IT media, research and exposition company. Founded in 1964, IDG had 1997 revenues of $2.05 billion and has more than 9,000 employees worldwide. IDG offers the widest range of media options that reach IT buyers in 75 countries representing 95% of worldwide IT spending. IDG's diverse product and services portfolio spans six key areas including print publishing, online publishing, expositions and conferences, market research, education and training, and global marketing services. More than 90 million people read one or more of IDG's 290 magazines and newspapers, including IDG's leading global brands — Computerworld, PC World, Network World, Macworld and the Channel World family of publications. IDG Books Worldwide is one of the fastest-growing computer book publishers in the world, with more than 700 titles in 36 languages. The "...For Dummies®" series alone has more than 50 million copies in print. IDG offers online users the largest network of technology-specific Web sites around the world through IDG.net (http://www.idg.net), which comprises more than 225 targeted Web sites in 55 countries worldwide. International Data Corporation (IDC) is the world's largest provider of information technology data, analysis and consulting, with research centers in over 41 countries and more than 400 research analysts worldwide. IDG World Expo is a leading producer of more than 168 globally branded conferences and expositions in 35 countries including E3 (Electronic Entertainment Expo), Macworld Expo, ComNet, Windows World Expo, ICE (Internet Commerce Expo), Agenda, DEMO, and Spotlight. IDG's training subsidiary, ExecuTrain, is the world's largest computer training company, with more than 230 locations worldwide and 785 training courses. IDG Marketing Services helps industry-leading IT companies build international brand recognition by developing global integrated marketing programs via IDG's print, online and exposition products worldwide. Further information about the company can be found at www.idg.com.   1/26/00

Author's Acknowledgments

From Betsy:

I wish to thank my husband, Mark, for encouraging me to take on this project. I've often joked that his idea of physical fitness is bending twice at the waist before we play tennis, but I'm proud that he's in incredible shape.

Thanks to Mark Reiter of IMG Literary for conceiving the book, as well as the fine folks at IDG Books Worldwide: Stacy Collins, Lisa Roule, and Gregg Summers.

I enjoyed being paired with my writing doubles partner, Mike Yorkey, who did a great job incorporating my thoughts and performing the bulk of the research. Without him on board, I would not have considered the project. Mike has written nearly two dozen books and is the former editor of *Focus on the Family* magazine. He and I will be teaming up on *In His Court*, which will be released in 2001.

Special thanks to experts who gave freely of their advice: Dr. Jim Loehr, a longtime friend; Fred Dolan of StretchMate; and David Donatucci, the director of the International Performance Institute at the Bollettieri Sports Academy in Bradenton, Florida.

Pamela Smith, a neighbor of mine, receives my thanks for granting permission to quote from her "Ten Commandments of Great Nutrition." Pam is a nationally known nutritionist, author, and culinary consultant whose most recent book is *The Diet Trap*.

Steven Mercer, my massage therapist, and fitness expert Dave Herman were a superb help with the photo illustrations, which were taken at The Fitness Center in Celebration, Florida, where Gar Simers is the general manager.

My thanks go to Dr. Bernard Watkin, Dr. Richard Steadman, Topper Haggerman, and John Adkins, who have helped me rebound from surgeries and injuries over the years.

I appreciate the insights of Alan Freedman and Joey Abramson (owners of six Fitness Outlet stores on the West Coast), Lisa Hutchison and Katrina Boyd of Ribet (a San Diego fitness retail company), and Chelsea Valach of Adventure 16 Outdoor and Travel Outfitters in Solana Beach, California.

Finally, a special note of appreciation is extended to my "readers" who provided insights on how to improve this manuscript: David and Jill Schmicherko, Loren Kurz, Lynette Winkler, and Nicole Yorkey.

Publisher's Acknowledgments

We're proud of this book; please register your comments through our IDG Books Worldwide Online Registration Form located at http://my2cents.dummies.com.

Some of the people who helped bring this book to market include the following:

*Acquisitions, Editorial, and
Media Development*

Project Editor: Gregg Summers

Acquisitions Editor: Stacy S. Collins

Copy Editors: Ellen Considine,
Gwenette Gaddis, Andrea Boucher

Acquisitions Coordinator: Lisa Roule

Technical Editor: Loren Kurz

Permissions Editor: Carmen Krikorian

Editorial Manager: Jennifer Ehrlich

Editorial Assistant: Jennifer Young

Production

Project Coordinator: Leslie Alvarez

Layout and Graphics: Clint Lahnen,
Brent Savage, Jacque Schneider,
Julia Trippetti, Brian Torwelle

Proofreaders: Corey Bowen, Mary Lagu,
Susan Moritz, Charles Spencer

Indexer: David Heiret

Photographer: Peter Barrett

General and Administrative

IDG Books Worldwide, Inc.: John Kilcullen, CEO; Bill Barry, President and COO

IDG Books Consumer Reference Group

Business: Kathleen A. Welton, Vice President and Publisher; Kevin Thornton, Acquisitions Manager

Cooking/Gardening: Jennifer Feldman, Associate Vice President and Publisher

Education/Reference: Diane Graves Steele, Vice President and Publisher; Greg Tubach, Publishing Director

Lifestyles: Kathleen Nebenhaus, Vice President and Publisher; Tracy Boggier, Managing Editor

Pets: Dominique De Vito, Associate Vice President and Publisher; Tracy Boggier, Managing Editor

Travel: Michael Spring, Vice President and Publisher; Suzanne Jannetta, Editorial Director; Brice Gosnell, Managing Editor

IDG Books Consumer Editorial Services: Kathleen Nebenhaus, Vice President and Publisher; Kristin A. Cocks, Editorial Director; Cindy Kitchel, Editorial Director

IDG Books Consumer Production: Debbie Stailey, Production Director

IDG Books Packaging: Marc J. Mikulich, Vice President, Brand Strategy and Research

The publisher would like to give special thanks to Patrick J. McGovern,
without whom this book would not have been possible.

◆

Contents at a Glance

Cartoons at a Glance

By Rich Tennant

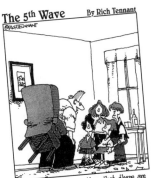

page 7

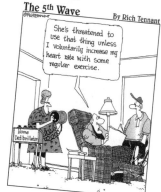

page 71

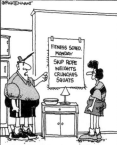

page 135

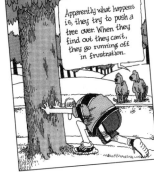

page 235

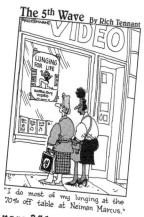

page 291

Fax: 978-546-7747
E-mail: richtennant@the5thwave.com
World Wide Web: www.the5thwave.com

Table of Contents

Introduction

∙∙

*O*ur generation isn't as fit as it used to be. Remember the jogging craze of the late 1970s? Remember how we baby boomers were going to be the fittest generation to walk the face of this earth?

Well, something happened along the way — golf. Sorry, I'm kidding, but as many 40-year-olds celebrated their "over-the-hill" parties with black crepe and funny cards, we stopped exercising. We became as sedentary as our parents did — something we promised ourselves that we would never do.

That, I believe, is not the way to go through life. Our bodies can remain quite fit for eight decades or longer. If you sew exercise and fitness into your life, you will reap the benefits of good health and longevity, even if you have fallen off the fitness bandwagon. In this book, I provide the essential info — the straight scoop in everyday English — that you absolutely need to know in order to get fit and stay fit in your forties and beyond. You won't find much, if any, jargon in this book because plain talk is what you need to hear on a topic that has lifelong implications. You *will* find tons of information presented in a fun, engaging way that won't make you feel guilty because you aren't quite as fit as you want to be. I think you'll find that *Fit Over 40 For Dummies* is a resource that you can return to time after time.

About This Book

This book is meant to be a reference. You can read it from cover to cover and discover the most important things you need to know about fitness in the middle-age years. You can skip around and read what looks interesting to you. Or you can turn to the index or table of contents and see exactly where to locate the information you need to know, complete with cross references to related topics you may want to brush up on.

Each chapter is divided into sections, and each section contains a piece of information about some important part of staying fit over 40. Things like this:

✔ How to determine your current fitness level.

✔ Tips for finding the best time and place to work out.

✔ Which home fitness equipment would be best for you.

    ✔ Guidelines for eating right.

    ✔ Advice on how to dress while working out.

    ✔ Ways to work out at work.

    ✔ Sample step-by-step exercise routines.

    ✔ How to prevent injuries while you exercise.

Foolish Assumptions

In writing this book, I've made some assumptions about you:

✔ You realize that you've been given only one body, and how you take care of that body can determine your quality of life from here on out.

✔ You know that you're on the "back nine" of life, and while you still have a bit of time before you reach the finishing holes, you'd rather play in good shape, not in poor shape.

✔ You don't want to become an expert on fitness. Instead, you just want to learn the basics about getting fit in ways that make sense for this busy period of life, which usually includes raising children and taking on added responsibility at work.

How This Book Is Organized

To help you find the information you need or are most interested in, this book is divided into five parts. Here's a rundown of each:

Part 1: Getting Started

In this part, I give you all the information you need to start a fitness program. I also explain why it's important to know your fitness level *before* you get started and how to set clear, specific goals. You can self-test your fitness in less than ten minutes at home with a quick, four-step program, or you can undergo a complete physical and treadmill test.

You will also learn how the body changes in the middle-age years so you won't be caught flat-footed by slower metabolism, menopause, or osteoporosis. You'll learn how fitness can reduce stress and even improve your sex life! I'll discuss the hidden benefits of fitness and cover some of the bases regarding diet and nutrition.

Part II: Exploring Your Options

This part will help you get familiar with the different types of exercise equipment and choose where to work out: in a fitness center, at work at an on-site gym, or at home. You'll also get valuable pointers on buying exercise equipment for your home.

This part also introduces the idea that fitness is really a three-legged stool — with cardiovascular exercise, strength training, and stretching each taking a leg. The foundation of your fitness program is probably going to be aerobic or cardiovascular exercise such as walking, jogging, or using treadmills or stationary bikes at your health club. But I'll explain why you can't overlook strength training with dumbbells, barbells, and weight machines like Nautilus.

Part III: Exercising for Life

This section starts by explaining why the first step to a good workout begins the night before — with a good night's rest. Then, to help you dress the part of a serious exerciser, you will learn about the new high-tech materials in workout wear, some of which prevent sweat from soaking your tops and leggings. This part also helps you choose the right shoes for your type of workout.

This part will also take you step-by-step through a series of exercises that you're welcome to adopt or adapt to your fitness plan. You can thumb through a special warm-up "protocol" designed by the trainers at the International Physical Institute in Bradenton, Florida, and then look through a pictorial essay of stretching exercises. This part also has two chapters outlining a series of lower-body and upper-body exercises that you can do on strength-training machines.

This section also provides tips on preventing and treating injuries and a reminder to cool down and drink plenty of water or Gatorade.

Part IV: Expanding Your Repertoire

If you're more into sports than exercises, this part has a chapter for you. What sport are you going to choose for "your" exercise? I'll discuss the various benefits and drawbacks of everything from walking and cycling to tennis and golf.

This part also introduces you to several sporting activities that weren't even around when you were growing up, such as in-line skating, mountain biking, snowboarding, rock climbing, and Tae-Bo. I have also devoted a chapter to some unique ways to work out: yoga, tai chi, and Pilates. Finally, you'll love the chapter on massage therapy, which extols the health benefits of masseuses kneading your tired muscles and aching joints after a fitness foray.

Part V: The Part of Tens

This part is designed to be a little more light-hearted than the others, but just as useful. You'll learn about great things exercise can do for you, some extreme and not-to-extreme sports you can try (just once) in your lifetime, motivational sports-related films you can rent on video, popular fitness magazines and Web sites you can check out, and interesting quotes on health and fitness.

Conventions and Icons Used in This Book

Because this book is designed to serve as a reference that you can use quickly and easily over and over again, some information is formatted so that it is easy for you to find and remember:

- *Italics*: Key phrases or terms are set in *italic* type, and they are defined within the next sentence or two.
- **Bold:** A few words of introductory **bold** type will give you a quick summary of the main idea of each item in some bulleted lists. (Don't know what a bulleted list is? You're reading one.)
- `Monofont`: Addresses that you are supposed to type into your Web browser to access Web sites are set in an easily recognizable type style called `monofont`.

Throughout this book, I also offset some information with attention-getting icons. When you see an icon, you will know what type of information is coming and that it deserves to be singled out. Here's what each icon will point out to you:

Points you should easily recall as you embark on a fitness program.

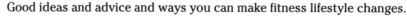

Good ideas and advice and ways you can make fitness lifestyle changes.

Useful, honest-to-goodness facts and figures about health and fitness.

 Cautions about common exercise mistakes or other things that could hurt your body, your ego, or your pocketbook.

 Stories from my tennis career or personal anecdotes or insights that may be useful to you. You can learn from some of my mistakes!

Where to Go from Here

Ready to leave the starting line? Not sure where the starting line is? No problem. If you don't know where to begin or need some motivation, the best place to start is with Part I. For those who've already resolved to become fitter, Part II will help you choose where to work out and understand why you need exercise that raises your heart rate and strengthens your muscles. Specific exercises are pictured in Part III.

If you already have a steady fitness program but are looking for ways to keep things fresh, then Part IV will plant plenty of new fitness ideas. But you can bounce all over this book. If you're interested in particular topics, head to the Table of Contents or the Index to find information quickly. Or just keep thumbing through pages until you find something that interests you; if you're interested in getting fit, it shouldn't take long!

Part I
Getting Started

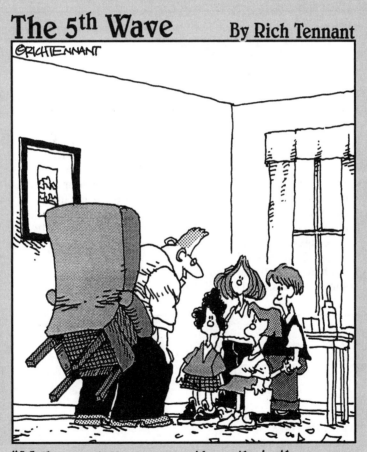

The 5th Wave   By Rich Tennant

"Well you tell your mother that there are no indications that I need to lose weight."

In this part . . .

Making an effort to trade a sedentary lifestyle for one that contains physical activity can turn back the hands of your body clock. Yes, aging is inevitable, but there's no reason why you can't feel years younger if you consistently exercise two, three, or four times a week, using short-term and long-term goals to inspire you.

This part explains why you should exercise in your middle-age years and gives you pointers on fitting fitness into your busy schedule. You'll also find out how your body changes with the passage of years and why nutrition becomes more important as we grow older and our metabolism slows. And you'll discover one boring, unchangeable truth: If you want to lose weight, you should eat less and exercise more.

Chapter 1

So, You Want to Get Fit

*O*ne thing all of us can agree on about life in our forties and beyond is this: *We're busy.* Careers are in full bloom, the kids are more involved than ever with school and extracurricular activities, and we are always finding some new project to volunteer our time for. (Resurrecting your "date night" with your partner to maintain a close connection would be nice as well.)

Something has to give. In your schedule, the first task you eliminate to save time is your plan to exercise. Once you cross off exercise from your to-do list, you're left with three choices:

1. Play the martyr and pretend you don't really need to exercise.

2. Figure there's always tomorrow and that you'll get around to exercising next week, next month, or next year.

3. Try again to find ways to include much-needed exercise time in your over-scheduled life.

The best alternative, of course, is the third choice. You can play the martyr or promise yourself that tomorrow is the start day, but those options aren't going to do you any good. Choosing to go through the rest of your days on earth without exercising means choosing a shortened life span and a lower quality of living. I implore you to do something *while you still can.* The fact that you are holding *Fit Over 40 For Dummies* in your hands is a great sign. Perhaps something prompted you to pick up this title at the bookstore or you received it as a gift. Either way, deep down you know that you're not as fit as you could be — or *should be.* Sure, you've added weight over the years, but you chalked up that weight gain to the passage of time. You've told yourself that putting on pounds as you grow older is as inevitable as retirement.

Well, I have some news for you: You *can* feel as fit as a fiddle — like you did 20 years ago. That's right. If you make the effort to trade your sedentary lifestyle for one that contains the crucial component — physical activity — there's no reason why you can't turn back the hands of your body clock.

I concede that aging is inevitable, and yes, we're all going to die. But those facts don't mean you have to shuffle into old age as a hunchback with a cane, looking for the nearest park bench to sit down on. After interviewing dozens of fitness experts over the years, I am convinced you can feel ten, 15, even 20 years younger than the birth date on your driver's license.

Allow me to expand on this point: If you are in your early forties, you can feel as fit as you did when you were in your mid-twenties; if you are in your late fifties, there's no reason why you can't match the physical fitness you enjoyed on the first anniversary of your 39th birthday. No, you won't ever measure up to the fitness peak you enjoyed during your late adolescence, but you can reclaim lost years if you start exercising today.

Yes, it's too bad that you're older, but as my fellow tennis compatriot Jimmy Connors once said, "It sure beats the alternative." Be thankful you're alive! Like all of us, you have much to live for: your family and children, your immediate family, your children's children (for you grandparents out there), close friends, wonderful careers, interesting hobbies, and inspirational travel to incredible places and locales you've yet to visit.

Years of maturation teach you what life is all about — the soft tenderness of the one we love till death do us part, the affectionate embrace of a child, and the chance to make a difference in other people's lives. "Youth is wasted on the young," said playwright George Bernard Shaw many years ago, and he was 100 percent correct. Use your maturity and experience to realize that *now* is the time to climb aboard the fitness bandwagon.

Making the Commitment Today

You begin by making a commitment to start exercising regularly. By regularly, I mean three days a week for five minutes a day. Yes, I said five minutes a day. That's all the time that you need to dedicate to start. Then you can look at increasing your exercise to 15 minutes a day, followed by a half-hour. Fifteen years ago, while I was playing tennis on the women's professional tour, I made a commitment to exercise consistently; since then I've exercised five days a week for at least one hour a day. You won't have to exercise as much as I do, but you must devise an exercise plan and stick to it.

People stop working out because they don't see immediate results. Perhaps that mindset can be attributed to the fast-paced "gotta have it now" society we live in, where 56K dial-up modems are dismissed as dinosaur connections to the Internet. You are spoiled with the swift efficiency of everything from PCs to jet travel to microwave ovens.

But physical fitness doesn't work that way. Fitness takes patience and perseverance, energy and enthusiasm, as well as sacrifices and spontaneity. Let this book inspire you to make specific changes in your lifestyle. Begin by sketching out a plan of action. Then act on that plan.

Perhaps you purchased this book as part of a New Year's resolution to embark on a fitness program. If so, I congratulate you. The New Year is a great time to resolve to change, because you mentally start with a clean slate. You can revamp your priorities and write "Work Out Today" on your personal calendar. If you have made your mind up to get in shape this New Year, let me encourage you to hold fast to your commitment. After all, plenty of people in their twilight years have wished they could wind back the hands of time. "Oh, if I had only known!" they say. "I would have done something about my fitness while I still could have."

Remember, though, that *any* time of year is a good time to start getting in better shape. It's never too late to become physically fit!

> *"The more sand that has escaped from the hourglass of our life, the clearer we should see through it."*
>
> —Jean-Paul Sartre

You still have many years left, but the grains of sand continue to pass through the hourglass. If you're fortunate to be healthy, albeit out of shape, count your blessings. Don't waste any more time thinking about your waist; now is the time to do something about it. The time to get off your duff is now! Nobody, while lying on their deathbed, has ever said, "I wish I spent less time exercising."

Overcoming the objections

Most people want to work out, but many lose their resolve. Many join a health club, but few stay very long. The reason is that the mind has an amazing ability to rationalize and create a long list of excuses so absurd that we dare not whisper them to our best friends.

Consider this litany of excuses not to exercise that you might have found yourself using at one time or another. I've included counterpoints for your reading pleasure:

✔ **Excuse**: It's too early in the morning.

   Counterpoint: It's too early for what? Not for the birds. Get up earlier.

✔ **Excuse**: I just ate.

   Counterpoint: All the more reason to walk it off. After-dinner walks can be the best, especially with a family member.

✔ **Excuse**: I'm too fat.

(continued)

(continued)

Counterpoint: You'll weigh less if you keep exercising regularly.

✔ **Excuse**: It's too cold.

Counterpoint: Dress warmly if you're walking or jogging outside. Most people work out at their homes or gyms, which are almost always heated.

✔ **Excuse**: It's too hot.

Counterpoint: Exercise early or late in the day, or exercise indoors. I doubt you could find a fitness center without air conditioning in this day and age.

✔ **Excuse**: I feel like sitting.

Counterpoint: The more you sit, the more you want to sit. Get going!

✔ **Excuse**: I'm too tired.

Counterpoint: Exercise will give you energy. You'll feel better when you're done. I guarantee it.

✔ **Excuse**: The treadmill hurts my knees.

Counterpoint: Then ride a recumbent bike or swim.

✔ **Excuse**: I don't have the right shoes.

Counterpoint: Sneakers are inexpensive. Buy new ones. You don't have to spend $100.

✔ **Excuse**: It's dark outside when I come home from work. I don't want to take a walk.

Counterpoint: Wear some reflective materials and carry a flashlight.

✔ **Excuse**: I'm afraid of dogs.

Counterpoint: Carry an old golf club. No dog will attack a crazy, club-wielding exercise fanatic.

✔ **Excuse**: It hurts to walk.

Counterpoint: Does it hurt to go five steps or 10 steps? Start with five steps and increase to 10 steps tomorrow. By the end of the week, you might be up to 20 steps. In no time, you can walk a mile in your shoes.

✔ **Excuse**: I'd rather go out to eat at a restaurant.

Counterpoint: Then park a mile or two from the restaurant and walk there. You'll work up a great appetite along the way.

✔ **Excuse**: I'm out of shape.

Counterpoint: So? A thousand-mile journey begins with a single step.

✔ **Excuse**: I can't leave the kids home alone.

Counterpoint: Many gyms offer some form of child care. Pay a teenager a few dollars to watch your children. Swap babysitting with a friend. Say you'll watch her kids when she exercises or runs errands. You can also walk or jog and have the kids ride their bikes alongside. You can also push your toddler in a baby jogger.

✔ **Excuse**: My husband won't join me.

Counterpoint: Let him loaf. You can't let a reluctant exerciser affect *your* health. Setting a good example, however, may inspire him to join you.

✔ **Excuse**: There's something good on TV.

Counterpoint: Then tape the show with your VCR.

✔ **Excuse**: I have only 20 minutes.

Counterpoint: Not only is that enough time, it's far better than doing nothing.

✔ **Excuse**: I'm on vacation.

Counterpoint: What better time to exercise than when you have so much free time?

Walking is a great travel pastime, especially if you're visiting the European crown cities.

✔ **Excuse:** I hate gardening.

Counterpoint: Then you're missing out on a great form of exercise.

✔ **Excuse:** I love shopping.

Counterpoint: Then make it a walking excursion!

✔ **Excuse:** I can come up with more reasons not to exercise.

Counterpoint: I'm sure you can. That still doesn't let you off the hook.

Setting Realistic Goals You Can Live With

Starting your exercise program means setting realistic goals — long-term and short-term benchmarks for things you want to accomplish in your life. (Don't worry. You have plenty of years left to set long-term goals. I still laugh when I recall Arnold Palmer's famous quip about turning 70 years old: "You know, I'm at an age where I don't even buy green bananas anymore.")

Short-term goals, when realistic, can motivate you to keep exercising for the long haul. Here are some examples of short-term goals:

✔ Walk 30 minutes without stopping.

✔ Walk one hour without stopping.

✔ Shovel your driveway clear of snow without overexerting yourself.

✔ Lose ten pounds.

✔ Wear older clothes that didn't fit.

✔ Quit smoking.

✔ Drink less alcohol.

Look at some long-term goals:

✔ Exercise consistently for the next 12 months.

✔ Lose 25 pounds.

✔ Lose 50 pounds.

✔ Drop one or two dress sizes.

- ✔ Wear size 34 pants again.

- ✔ Run in a 10-kilometer race.

- ✔ Lower your blood pressure.

- ✔ Play in a father-son tennis tournament.

- ✔ Hike to the top of Pikes Peak (or some other mountain or hill in your region).

- ✔ Ski six straight days in Utah.

- ✔ Go on a New England bicycle tour in the fall.

Ask yourself what short-term or long-term goals appeal to you. Goal setting is important because it shows that you are serious about improving your physical fitness.

Here are the short-term goals I think you should set *for your exercise program*:

1. Work out three days a week. Whether it's for five or 50 minutes, three days a week is your baseline.

2. Add five to ten minutes to your thrice-a-week workouts during the first two weeks.

3. Be at 30 minutes, three times a week, by the end of your third week.

4. Maintain this exercise level for several months.

5. Add a fourth day to your weekly exercise plan after you reach the six-month point, or anytime along the way.

Okay, what you've just read is fairly safe stuff that you could read in a thousand other fitness books. What I'm about to suggest is something revolutionary, and it's this: *Try to exercise every day.*

Don't kid yourself. If you promise yourself that you are going to exercise two, three days a week, life has a way of erasing one of those days each week. If you make a commitment to exercise *every* day — which could mean a 6 a.m. visit every morning to your fitness club, a 30-minute walk during your lunch break, riding a stationary bike after dinner, or strolling through a nearby park on the weekend — you should have no problem exercising at least *four* days a week. In other words, if you shoot for seven days a week, you should be able to get in four or five exercise periods.

Research has shown that working out once a week is like spinning your wheels in the mud — you won't get anywhere. Some fitness gains are made when you exercise intensely twice a week. Thrice is nice: Three or four exercise sessions will greatly improve your fitness level. But five or six exercise periods move up your fitness level in ways that appear to be revolutionary. And more frequent workouts speed up fat loss. Keep that thought in mind if you're searching for inspiration.

Because the general rule says that it takes 21 days to establish a new habit, you need to give yourself a chance to change things around. Write your exercise appointments in your daily calendar and dare yourself to scratch them out.

Finding the Right Time to Exercise

I know you are expecting me to say that morning is the best time to exercise. While the early hours of the day are the preferred time (the best reason being that you can't cancel a workout that you've already finished), it's not the only time. The best time to exercise is *when it works for you.*

Because your body is capable of exercising at any hour, you can exercise any time of day (or night). Shawn Fanning, the creator of Napster (the controversial Web site that allows computer users to trade digital music files), lifts weights after 11 p.m. at a 24-Hour Fitness outlet in Silicon Valley; that time is what works in his busy schedule. I heard about a morning DJ in Texas who sets his alarm for 4 a.m. so he can run and lift weights before his drive-time shift; that exercising schedule may sound crazy, I know, but it works for him. If you're a light sleeper who's raring to go at 4:30 a.m., get up and go! If you're a night owl who gets a second wind at 10 p.m., huff and puff then. Only you know what's best for you.

Having said that, I must remind you that incorporating exercise into your *morning* schedule is better because the longer you go through the day without exercise, the easier it becomes to say, "I'm tired. *Manana.*"

One study tracked exercisers for a year to see how long they followed through on their commitment to get in shape. Seventy-five percent of those who exercised in the morning were still exercising a year later. Half of those who worked out at noontime stayed with the program, but only 25 percent of those who exercised in the evening maintained their exercise regimen.

Conclusion: Mornings are best, and then you can rest.

Flexing at dawn: Early morning workouts

If you're going to start working out at dawn, you should know that just before you awake, the body's core temperature is around 97 degrees. Although you may feel warm when you awake, your body's temperature naturally decreases as you sleep. Because your body's thermostat is set on low in the dawn's early hours, you probably don't feel like jumping out of bed and jumping rope for ten minutes. This low body temperature explains why some people do not even want to *think* about working out or performing any physical activity until they drink their second cup of coffee. Many folks rather enjoy the calming effect that the morning brings.

Early morning exercise may be the answer to your workday blahs and may make you feel better than any second cup of coffee. That's why I recommend that you take a walk or visit the gym early one day, even if you're not a morning person. You may discover that you rather enjoy the circulation boost and endorphin rush you get from early morning fitness. Soon you may crave the feel-good sensation that early morning workouts give your body.

Here are some tips you can employ to help you keep your a.m. exercise appointment:

- **Call your exercise buddy the night before.** Many people find that exercising with a friend is more fun than going it alone, and the two of you can motivate and encourage each other to greater fitness heights (see "Taking your pulse with a pal" in this chapter). Nobody likes getting stood up, however, so a friendly phone call the evening before will be a reminder to both of you that tomorrow's the day!

- **Pack your exercise clothing ahead of time.** When you're exercising before work, every ten minutes count. You avoid rushing to pack everything at the last minute if you get your clothes in order the night before. Arriving at the fitness gym only to realize that you forgot your sneakers or new underwear can be pretty frustrating. Also, you can bet that your sleeping spouse or partner appreciates your courtesy in not fumbling around, looking for your jock strap in the dark.

- **Pack your breakfast and lunch the night before.** You should wait 90 minutes after a big meal before working out. So prepare to eat after your workout by packing your food the night before. Again, preparation means one less thing to do in the morning. (Morning exercisers should, however, eat a little something before their workout — a piece of fruit or toast or some yogurt — to jump-start their system.)

- **Set two alarms.** Don't ask me why, but Murphy's Law (anything that can go wrong will go wrong) reigns supreme at 5:45 a.m. — alarms fail to go off or people sleep through several "snooze" segments. Setting a second alarm across the room means you actually have to get out of bed to turn the darn thing off. Then you're awake.

Shaping up at noon or the end of the day: Tips for 9-to-5 exercisers

Try as I might, I'm sure I won't be able to convince everybody to become morning exercisers. Some people simply cannot get enough motivation to work out then, and family commitments or extra-long commutes may make working out just too difficult in the morning. For those of you who just must wait until later in the day to exercise, here are some pointers for keeping that workout appointment with yourself:

- **Work smart.** There's an old saying: "Work expands to fill the time." In other words, if you schedule two hours for a meeting that can be wrapped up in 60 minutes, you and the group will take exactly 120 minutes to accomplish your business. If you are in a leadership position, announce your intention to end the meeting in one hour (especially if it's an 11 a.m. meeting and you want to work out over lunchtime, or it's 4 p.m. and this is the last meeting of the day).

- **Try to arrive just a little before noon.** If you're able to exercise at a corporate fitness facility or a nearby health club, arriving five or ten minutes before the noon rush may be the difference between finding an empty treadmill or getting aced out. You can also get on your favorite strength-training machines without having to wait or bounce around to different machines.

- **If you're exercising right after work, make it work for you.** The easiest time to cancel a physical activity is at the end of the workday. You're tired, stressed out, and worried about how much you have to do. You know that family activities and responsibilities are waiting for you at home. But if you can leave work on time, get your workout in, and arrive home in time for dinner, you're going to feel a *lot* better. You have to be disciplined to get your tasks done, keep that appointment you made with yourself (and your exercise buddy), and put something into your fitness time. Exercising gets easier each time you stay with the program, however.

- **Finally, know that all is not lost if you don't exercise before dinner.** Although not ideal, you can still exercise in the several hours between dinner and bedtime. A long walk with your partner, for instance, provides great fitness benefits and gives the two of you an opportunity to catch up and share how your day went.

BETSY'S RACKET

Working out motherhood

Becoming a mother at the age of 41 forced me to become more organized with my life. I used to let the day unfold and worked out when it was convenient, but becoming a mom changed all that.

Basically, my workouts revolve around Maggie's nap times. I loved doing my fitness regimen when Maggie took her morning nap. Now that she's older, she doesn't nap in the a.m. and I've had to adjust to having one less time window open to work out. The day will come when Maggie no longer naps at all, and that day will be fine with me. If I have to find someone to babysit Maggie for an hour or two so that I can do my fitness work, I'll organize it. If I have to get in treadmill time after 9 p.m. when she's gone to bed, I'll make the adjustment.

Staying with Your Program

Another important aspect of fitness is consistency. The way you develop consistency is by scheduling a set time to exercise. This step sounds so simple that an elementary-age child can follow it, but I know how hard it is to bring consistency to our busy and always-changing lives.

Human nature, being what it is, dictates that if something is not scheduled in the calendar book, you're going to skip it. An appointment with yourself to exercise is often the easiest thing to drop from an overburdened schedule. Besides, when you're exhausted after a long day, working out and making yourself even *more* tired is the last thing you want to do.

Rewarding your own good behavior

David Donatucca, a personal trainer who directs the International Performance Institute in Bradenton, Florida, remembers an executive named Susan who routinely canceled her appointments at the last minute. David heard all the excuses: "My meeting ran late . . . the boss needed to see me . . . my quarterly report was due . . . someone cornered me in the hall."

He racked his brain thinking of ways he could motivate Susan. She understood the benefits of exercise and, once she arrived at his gym, she put her heart and soul into her workouts. Getting her to the gym was the difficult part.

Then David had an idea. "Susan, why don't you try this," he said. "Each time you work out with me, reward yourself. Set up a little jar and every time you go to the gym, put $20 in it."

Susan raised her eyebrows.

"Okay, make it $5," said David. "After a few months, splurge on something that you usually wouldn't purchase for yourself: maybe a new briefcase, a new sport coat, a set of CDs, or a Walkman for your workouts. Treat yourself."

Susan began rewarding herself after every workout. David never heard what she purchased for herself, but whatever she bought with her reward money was icing on the cake.

A reward system makes exercise a positive experience. Usually, everybody only listens to negative self-talk when it comes to exercise:

✔ If you don't work out, you're doomed to an early grave.

✔ If you don't work out, you become such a couch potato that walking to the mailbox qualifies as a major workout.

Turn negative self-talk around by thinking about the rewards of working out. Remind yourself of how good you feel about yourself. Keep in mind that you are paying *yourself* to keep your exercise appointments. Tell your spouse that both of you will dine at your favorite restaurant if you stay with your exercise program for one month. Or enjoy a long weekend out of town as a three-month reward. Exercise shouldn't be seen as a punishment or the price you have to pay for just living. Exercise should be a benefit to you.

Taking your pulse with a pal

Let me be honest: You're less likely to break an exercise appointment if you made it with a friend — especially if the scheduled time is a 6:15 a.m. rendezvous at the neighborhood fitness center. Nobody wants to let a friend down — or get razzed for sleeping in.

Working out with a friend gives you someone to talk to. Instead of chatting over a café mocha at Starbucks, you and your friend can laugh, swap stories, and share interesting details about your lives as you stair step on side-by-side machines. You can exchange hot stock tips as you pound the treadmills or take turns pushing plates on the Nautilus machines.

Some forms of exercise *must* be done with a friend. It takes two to play tennis, of course. A hot racquetball game with a worthy opponent burns calories. Long walks always go better with company (except on those occasions when you prefer solitude). Ask one of your best friends to join you, no matter what the physical activity is. She may have been waiting for your call all along! Together, you can push each other to keep on keeping on.

Chapter 2

Oh, My Aching Bones: What Happens When the Body Ages

*I*t's enough to give you a panic attack, the way the body changes in your forties, fifties, and sixties. When you throw in major shifts in your attitude and some emotional upheaval, the midlife years can prompt a classic midlife crisis. You need to have an idea of the physical changes that are coming so you won't be blindsided by them. These changes are natural and come with maturity — they are not necessarily indications of a disease you may contract or a loss of ability you may experience in the future. Knowledge can be reassuring. Take a look at some of the natural physical changes you can expect from your body.

Marking Time: Signs of Aging

No doubt — you *look* older when you *are* older. As you travel the road of life, here are some freeway markers to look for:

- ✔ **Loss of hair.** Men may lose hair by the handfuls or watch their hairlines slowly recede; more than one-third of men show signs of male-pattern baldness after the age of 25.

- ✔ **Graying of hair.** Both sexes may contend with the graying of hair, especially in their fifties.

✔ **Crow's feet.** After years of squinting, you may develop these fine lines extending from the outer corners of your eyes.

✔ **Age spots.** Darkening age spots become more noticeable on the arms and face, depending on how much sun exposure you've endured over the years. (I call Florida my home, and prolonged sun exposure here turns residents into prunes — which is why I carefully slather gobs of sunscreen on my face and body.)

I concede that there is not much you can do to fight these cosmetic signs of aging, unless you submit yourself to expensive plastic surgery. I feel, however, that consistent exercise brings a radiance to your face, tones muscles, and reduces weight. Those benefits add up to a healthy body, which reflects a healthy person — young or old.

You can, however, have far more success holding off your aging body's tendency to slow down and gain weight if you exercise regularly.

Your sluggish metabolism

Metabolism is the chemical process that takes oxygen and food and alters those substances to fuel the growth, maintenance, and repair of your body. You stopped growing years ago, of course, so the food you eat (and oxygen you breathe in, to a lesser extent) is turned into the fuel the body needs merely to replenish itself.

You probably noticed that your metabolism has slowed down since you reached your forties. Let me paint a picture to describe the changes in your metabolism. Imagine yourself driving a cherry-red Corvette with a 5.7-liter V8 SFI engine. When you were young, that finely tuned engine roared to life. As the years pass, however, you don't take that car out as often. Your 'Vette has fallen into disuse, and the engine has sludge deposits. The car doesn't respond well when you slam the engine into gear and peel out. That car needs to be maintained and well-exercised to stay in top shape. Your body requires the same attention.

When your metabolism slows down, it affects five basic elements of physical fitness:

✔ Cardiovascular endurance

✔ Muscle endurance

✔ Muscle strength

✔ Flexibility

✔ Weight control

Accelerating your metabolism

You can turn your slowing metabolism process around through exercise. Look at the changes you can make by improving your metabolism:

- ✔ **Increased cardiovascular endurance.** Your metabolism provides the needed fuel to keep the heart running.

- ✔ **Improved muscle endurance, strength, and flexibility.** Your muscles are enhanced as a result of your muscle tissues being broken down, rested, and rebuilt by your metabolism.

- ✔ **Better weight control.** The role of your metabolism is self-evident. When your metabolism is raised through exercise, more calories are burned, which results in more weight loss.

Feeding your metabolism

Your body separates the calories you consume into three areas: carbohydrates, proteins, and fats. Your body needs all three substances to survive. Carbohydrates are basically the fuel that runs your body. Proteins build muscles, repair bones, and repair injuries. Fat insulates and protects the vital organs and is called upon for long-term energy.

Your metabolism is affected by your eating habits. In your middle-age years, you need fewer calories to maintain your weight, so you should eat less. In addition, *when* you eat is just as important as *what* you eat. You may want to consider eating smaller meals four, five, or six times a day instead of skipping breakfast, grabbing a quick lunch, and feasting on a big dinner. Eating smaller meals more often can stimulate faster metabolism and result in weight loss.

Don't skip breakfast! Many health authorities recommend eating a healthy breakfast, a moderate lunch, and a skimpy dinner (skip that evening snack) as a way to trim unwanted fat.

As for my eating schedule, I start off the morning by eating a big bowl of fruit. I was never a cereal eater, but if you are, that's fine — as long as you crunch down a cereal low in sugar and fat.

Pudding on the pounds

Like clockwork, as you age, you lose muscle mass. As you lose muscle mass, your metabolism slows. As your metabolism slows, you gain weight. As you gain weight, you tend to say, "Oh, heck with it, pass me the Pringles." For women, this weight gain settles in the lower body — hips, buttocks, and thighs. For men, it's the Michelin look — a tire wrapped around the midsection. Unless you're taking exercise countermeasures, you gain one to two pounds a year, even with a reduced food intake.

The top ten signs you're getting older

10. Everything hurts — and what doesn't hurt, doesn't work.

9. You're 17 around the neck, 42 around the waist, and 105 around the golf course.

8. Your back goes out more than you do.

7. Your arms are almost too short to read the newspaper.

6. Your knees buckle, but your belt won't.

5. When you do the Hokey Pokey, you put your left hip out — and it stays out.

4. You run out of breath walking *down* a flight of stairs.

3. No one expects you to run into a burning building.

2. Your joints are more accurate than the National Weather Service.

1. You quit trying to hold your stomach in, no matter who walks into the room.

Gaining weight is not harmful per se, you just don't want to gain *too much* weight (refer to Tables 3-4 and 3-5). Maintaining an acceptable weight results in numerous health benefits and places less stress on bones and joints.

People who tend to gain weight mostly in their hips and buttocks have "pear-shaped" figures; those who gain weight mostly in the abdomen have more of an "apple" shape. The distinction is important because apple-shaped people are at an increased risk for health problems associated with obesity — diabetes, coronary heart disease, and high blood pressure. Although you can't do anything to change your body type (it's all in your genes), you can still take steps to control your weight by eating nutritiously and exercising consistently.

Expiring after retiring

A surprising statistic: Your mortality rate is the highest in your life during the six months after retirement. You would think that kicking back and watching TV from the La-Z-Boy would be the *least* stressful thing you could do to a body, but the opposite is true. More people die just after retirement because all the stresses — physical and mental — suddenly shut down. Retirees don't have any obligations. Nothing hanging over their heads. No projects to get done by Tuesday. No exercise. Then kaboom! Retirees succumb to sudden heart attacks or lightning-quick illnesses that invade their bodies.

Conclusion: The kick-back years are the time to kick-start your exercise routine.

Find out if your body type is an apple or a pear by surfing the Web. Begin by searching for "apple or pear weight calculation." You'll be led to several sites that can calculate where most of the fat on your body is located.

Regarding Females

Nature is not kind to a woman's body as she passes through two significant stages of life unique to the gender — childbirth and menopause. In addition, physical changes begin taking place around 30 years of age: the start of a slow, steady decline in youthful muscle mass; and a slower metabolism rate that causes her to burn calories more slowly. You add up all these factors, and you can see why women have a tough time fighting middle-age spread.

Gaining weight after childbirth

The first significant change to a woman's body comes during pregnancy. Women's bodies have evolved to store the fat that they need to carry their baby to term and breast-feed. The average woman gains 25 to 35 pounds during pregnancy — pounds that have a way of permanently altering a woman's figure. Women are likely to remain ten to 20 pounds heavier after giving birth, and their bodies store about half the fat gained during pregnancy in the hips, thighs, and abdominal muscles.

After childbirth, many women experience a huge lifestyle change that comes with caring and nurturing their offspring. (In other words, no time to exercise.) For many new moms, the post-partum period is the first time they have actively tried to lose weight, and all too often those attempts bring limited success. That's why very few women can become pregnant, bring several children into this world, age gracefully into their forties and fifties, and still fit into their wedding dress. It's just not going to happen. Physical decline is inevitable, although some women are lucky enough to be born with fabulous genes. For many women, however, all they have to do is look at food and they gain weight.

May I offer an observation? If you never lost those post-pregnancy pounds and are still overweight, discuss the issue with your partner. Chances are he feels uncomfortable about raising the topic, because he knows weight is such a sensitive issue. What do you plan to do? Are you going to exercise more? How can your spouse help? Unless your husband is one of those unique individuals with washboard abs and buns of steels, you're both probably in the same weight and fitness class. Resolve to work out together. Following an exercise program and trimming pounds as a couple activity will bring you closer together. That closeness may be the best reward of all.

The "change of life"

No discussion of how a woman's body changes in the midlife years would be complete without a discussion of menopause. Today's aging female population — 21 million baby-boom women will reach menopause in the next ten years — has the "M" word on its mind. Menopause has been called the "change of life" for generations, because it marks the end of a woman's ability to bear children. In starker terms, menopause is the slow death of the ovaries and their ability to produce *ova,* or eggs. The average age a woman begins menopause is 51.4 years. The vast majority of women in their forties still await the onset of menopause. What happens in the meantime is that women enter a transitional period called *perimenopause,* which literally means "near menopause." Perimenopause usually begins in a woman's early forties and lasts an average of seven to ten years. During this period, the ovaries wax and wane before sputtering to a stop, signifying that menopause has begun.

The ovaries produce the primary hormones of estrogen and progesterone. As fewer and fewer of these hormones are released in the perimenopausal years, the female menstrual cycle takes a hit. Suddenly, three or four days are clipped off your four-week menstrual cycle or your five-day menstrual flow shortens to two days.

What troubles some women about menopause is the fact that they live in a youth-oriented culture. Menopause implies old age, and old age implies uselessness and mental deterioration. For many women, menopause signals an irreversible sign of aging and the start of the slow, inevitable march toward the end of life.

A little perspective is called for. Menopause may mean the end of a woman's ability to bear children, but it is far from the end of her life. Women's life expectancies have increased; women are living 30 to 35 years past menopause. Because women are enjoying longer lives, including plenty of exercise along the way may help to improve their quality of life during their advanced years.

As menopause nears, women begin experiencing wonderful events such as hot flashes, depression, dizziness, weight gain, headaches, sweating, and excitability. Exercise is one of the few tools you have to get through this difficult, once-in a-lifetime event.

Osteoporosis

Osteoporosis is a common disease that causes your bones to become porous and brittle later in life. This disease affects more than 10 million adults in the United States — mainly women — and females have a 25 percent chance of developing osteoporosis. Women reach peak bone mass by age 30, after which time bone mineral density starts declining. Dwindling estrogen amounts after menopause cause the bones to become thin and brittle. This bone-loss disease produces noticeable limps and hunched backs. I hurt when I see older women walking in a stoop because of their weakened spines.

Ironically, the best exercise to prevent osteoporosis is walking, because walking is a weight-bearing exercise. Jogging and jumping rope certainly fill the bill, as well. Gym workouts maintain and build bone mass and density, so don't be bashful about pushing plates on Nautilus machines. All of these exercises can boost bone density 3 to 5 percent a year in those adults who previously didn't exercise.

Many women consider estrogen replacement therapy (ERT). This form of therapy is not without its drawbacks, however. Before you begin ERT, you must thoroughly discuss the benefits and drawbacks with your doctor. Meanwhile, it never hurts to take calcium supplements — up to 1000 mg per day before menopause and up to 1500 mg after menopause. Milk (whole, 2 percent, and skim) is high in calcium, as are yogurt, cheese, vegetables, tofu, and calcium-fortified orange juice.

Male Menopause?

Men are not immune to hormonal, physiological, and chemical changes; their bodies also experience some transformations between the ages of 40 and 55. Some pop psychologists even have a name for it: male menopause.

Whether male menopause really exists is cause for debate in the medical world. Middle-aged men cannot disregard the physical changes sapping their energy levels, however, or their sagging bodies. Men experience varying degrees of lethargy, bouts of depression, and fluctuating mood swings during this time. The underlying reason why some medical professionals believe that males experience a change like menopause is due to the steady decline of *testosterone.* Testosterone is the hormone responsible for such male characteristics as a beard, body hair, and libido — as well as a muscular physique. From its height in late adolescence, testosterone production steadily and gradually declines about 1 percent a year.

Men should adjust their mental outlooks during their middle-age years. One of the best ways to adjust a sluggish attitude is through exercising. Many men, when their vital energies run down, pursue athletic activities less energetically and frequently. The *opposite* has to happen. Now is not the time to let it all go, but the time to go for it.

Raising Your Expectations: Preparing for a Longer Life

I was born in 1956, nearly smack dab in the middle of that cultural phenomenon known as the baby boom — children born between the years of 1946–64. I am part of the biggest generation in U.S. history — presently 76 million boomers are passing through the American scene.

If you are also a baby boomer, you cannot deny that you have grown older. You have reached the next stage of your life: middle age. Middle age offers a time of transition — when parents die and children leave the home. A time when fit bodies are replaced by sore backs and flabby midsections. A time when you receive your first AARP mailing. A time when you begin to think about the sunset years and retirement.

Living long and prospering

Wait a minute! You don't want to grow old. Old age is for . . . old people. Old age is gray hair and wrinkles and walkers and eating applesauce and shuffling slippered feet down a linoleum-tiled hall. Ah, but old age doesn't have to be that way, at least for a very long time. Yes, it's inevitable that you will grow old and die one day, but what influences the need for getting in shape now is the irrefutable fact that folks are living longer and longer. (See Table 2-1.)

People living at the dawn of the twentieth century lived with the strong possibility that they could be pushing up the daisies when they reached 45 years of age. One hundred years later, you find yourself living in a highly technological society with breakthrough medical advancements. You've been handed 30 extra years of life on a silver platter. With such a significant increase in the average life span, a healthy person in his or her middle-age years today can savor the fullness of life for many years to come.

Some of you crossing the threshold into middle age may hear that there's "a lot of will but no way." Don't you believe it. If you *think* you're getting old, you *act* accordingly. Because you've been handed this incredible gift — a relatively healthy life — aren't you dying (oops, wrong word) to live the rest of your days fit and sassy beyond your chronological age? I know I am.

No reason exists — barring an unforeseen disease or accidental catastrophe — that should keep you from enjoying a vibrant life until you are well into your seventies, even your eighties. I love what Moses said in Psalm 90:10: "The length of our days is seventy years — or eighty, if we have the strength." To "have the strength," you must take care of your body by exercising moderately, eating the right foods, and sleeping enough, among other things.

Table 2-1	Years of Life Expected at Birth, 1900-1995		
Year	*Male*	*Female*	*Both sexes*
1900	46.3	48.3	47.3
1910	48.4	51.8	50.0
1920	53.6	54.6	54.1
1930	58.1	61.6	59.7
1940	60.8	65.2	62.9
1950	65.6	71.1	68.2
1960	66.6	73.1	69.7
1970	67.1	74.7	70.8
1980	70.0	77.5	73.7
1990	71.8	78.8	75.4
1995	72.5	78.9	75.8

Source: National Center for Health Statistics (1999)

Time may be on your side

All this talk about baby boomers growing older sparked an interesting idea for a book: *RealAge: Are You Young as You Can Be?* (Cliff Street, 1999) by Michael F. Roizen, M.D. In his best-selling book, Dr. Roizen tells nail-biting boomers that they might not be as old as they think they are, which is a comforting proposition (and perhaps one reason his book hit a nerve).

At face value, Dr. Roizen's theory makes sense. All of us can think of people who look years older because of overwork, lack of exercise, and a poor diet taking their tolls. On the flip side, perpetual "sunny boys" or "gorgeous gals" flaunt slim, trim bodies and worker-bee movements as a testimony to living a healthy lifestyle. Perhaps you remember attending your 25-year high school reunion. All of your classmates were about 43 years of age chronologically, but did they all look the same age? Of course not. I was *shocked* to see the differences in my old classmates at Northeast High School in St. Petersburg, Florida, when I attended my reunion. My classmates didn't look the same age, because they *weren't* the same age — at least in biological and physiological terms.

As Dr. Roizen conducted his research, he saw age not as a chronological measurement, but as a measurement determined by the rate at which the cardiovascular and immune systems declined. While a person's chronological age is fixed, his biological age may be years older — or younger — depending on a number of factors.

Dr. Roizen and a team of scientists pored through 25,000 medical studies of how people age and what could be done to prevent aging. They found that 44 factors promote age reduction — which means you can do 44 different things to reduce your rate of aging. From that information, Dr. Roizen's team developed a RealAge survey that asks 125 detailed questions about a variety of behaviors related to aging. A sample of the questions:

✔ What is your blood pressure?

✔ How often do you eat breakfast each week?

✔ What is your heart rate?

✔ Does your weight fluctuate?

✔ How many minutes per week do you spend exercising?

✔ How many minutes per week do you do strength-building exercises?

✔ How many servings of fish do you eat a week?

✔ How many meals with tomato paste do you have each week?

✔ Do you floss your teeth?

✔ Do you own a dog?

Your answers either add time to your chronological age (for instance, high blood pressure adds three years) or subtract (low blood pressure subtracts three years).

Dr. Roizen adds that even lifestyle changes made in the middle-age years make a difference. For example, if you exercise a lot as a youngster but quit when you marry and begin raising a family, that early-in-life exercise shows no longevity benefit today. However, if you start exercising in your forties, fifties, and sixties — or even later — your body receives considerable benefits. Another reminder that it is never too late to start an exercise program.

You see, the natural progression of aging is accelerated by disuse. Stop exercising the muscles and your heart rate pushes up; the body begins to act older than its years. If you continue to work your cardiovascular system and muscles, your body rebounds and becomes very resilient. Jim Loehr, a sports psychologist and author of several fitness-related books, told me that he has seen 80-year-old men greatly increase their functionality after beginning a weight-training program — at their age! "Studies show that weight training by the elderly results in muscle tissue growth that is nearly as quick as that growth in 25-year-old men," said Jim. "The point is this: If you stimulate your muscles through exercise and weight training, they respond. But if you don't, the body thinks it's all over, and then it starts shutting down."

Jim uses himself as an example. When he was in his thirties, he couldn't run a six-minute mile if a winning Powerball ticket was waiting for him at the finish line. For that matter, he couldn't have finished a mile in eight minutes. Today at 57, Jim can run a six-minute mile. "I've reversed the aging process, which anyone can do at any time in life, depending on how much energy you put into it," he said.

TIP

Taking the RealAge test online

Would you like to discover your RealAge? It's just a few clicks away on RealAge.com, where you can calculate an accurate RealAge and receive personalized recommendations on how to become younger than your chronological years. Click on RealAge Test and spend around 10 to 15 minutes answering the questions. Be honest. Don't automatically answer "Excellent" to the question: "How would you rate your physical health compared to others at your chronological age?"

I took the test, which revealed that I am 37.5 in biological years. The results pleasantly surprised me and made me feel good. What the RealAge Test did was confirm that the lifestyle choices I've made over the years can slow and even reverse the rate of aging.

Ten ways you can reduce your RealAge

According to Dr. Michael Roizen, the following are just a few of the steps you can take to live longer:

1. **Be happily married.** It's a fact: Married men and women live longer than divorced people or those who never marry.

2. **Take your vitamins.** Dr. Roizen says taking vitamin C, vitamin E, calcium, vitamin D, folate, and vitamin B6 can make your RealAge six years younger.

3. **Eat lots of tomato sauce.** Men chowing down pizza, spaghetti, and other tomato-based sauces live longer, but tomato paste has no effect on women's life spans.

4. **Take hormone replacement therapy.** Women who take estrogen replacement therapy during their menopausal years have a RealAge eight years younger.

5. **Take your fill of sex.** The more you climax, the longer you live.

6. **Floss your teeth.** Mother was right — keeping your teeth and gums healthy can make your RealAge six years younger.

7. **Drink alcohol moderately.** The French must know something, because Dr. Roizen says that folks who drink one or two glasses of wine each day live longer.

8. **Don't skip breakfast.** The body needs fuel when you wake up.

9. **Eat your fruit and veggies.** You need at least four servings from each food group every day.

10. **Do all three components of physical activity.** Adopting a three-tiered exercise plan that includes burning calories, increasing stamina, and building strength can make your RealAge as much as nine years younger.

Chapter 3

Finding Out How Fit You Are Now

• •

In This Chapter

▶ Determining your fitness level

▶ Calculating your Body Mass Index (BMI)

▶ Determining your dimensions

▶ Examining your physical exam

• •

*N*ow that you're inspired to make fitness a lifestyle in your middle-age years, two things must be accomplished at this momentous moment:

1. Make a self-determination of how fit you are.

2. Receive a doctor's clearance by undergoing a medical exam.

Sizing Up Your Fitness Level

If you've been sleeping for 20 years like Rip Van Winkle and have awakened to the importance of fitness, I welcome you back. One of the first steps you must take is to figure out what shape you are in *right now*. My intention is not to depress you, but to give you a starting point or benchmark. After several months on your fitness program, this reference point enables you to look back and say, "Yes, I've come a long way."

Here are several ways to determine what shape you're in:

✔ Any **fitness center** worth its mission statement can assess your fitness level. Just ask for an assessment when you sign up. A staff member measures your resting heart rate, your heart rate under physical exertion, the number of push-ups and sit-ups you can do in a minute, strength on various exercise machines, and how long you can walk on a treadmill, among several other in-house tests.

✔ A **personal trainer**, at a gym or your house, can take the same measurements.

✔ A full-bore **treadmill test** can be performed at a sports medicine center. (These tests can be costly; check to see if your medical insurance covers these exams.) Speaking from personal experience, a complete treadmill test most accurately assesses your cardiovascular fitness level.

✔ **Self-administered tests,** like the ones I'm about to describe, are easy to perform and take just a few minutes. These tests, while not scientific, should give you a rudimentary idea where you stand on several components of overall fitness.

Test 1: Upper body

Count how many push-ups you can do in a minute. Note your ranking. Women may do modified push-ups by starting with their knees on the ground and slightly bent.

Rankings	Number of Push-Ups
Very fit	25
Average	15
Out of shape	7
Couch potato	less than 7

Test 2: Middle body

Lie down on your back. Cup your hands and place them behind your head. Do a half sit-up and hold your body at a 45-degree angle for as long as you can. If this exercise is a literal pain in the neck, stop immediately. Don't forget to note your ranking.

Rankings	Length of Endurance
Very fit	25 seconds
Average	15 seconds
Out of shape	7 seconds
Couch potato	less than 7 seconds

Test 3: Lower body

Skiers should be familiar with this exercise, which is great for developing strong leg muscles. Lean against a wall and "sit" against it with your legs bent at a 90-degree right angle. Hold this position for as long as you can. (You'll feel your legs burn.) Jot down your ranking.

Rankings	Length of Endurance
Very fit	90 seconds
Average	60 seconds
Out of shape	30 seconds
Couch potato	less than 30 seconds

Test 4: Flexibility

Before conducting this test, go for a five-minute walk and do some jumping jacks. Get loose and warm. Sit on the floor and place a yardstick between your legs so that the 15-inch mark measures up with the end of your feet (and the 1-inch mark is roughly between your knees). Your feet should be shoulder-width apart — about 10 inches. Slowly stretch forward and slide your fingertips along the yardstick as far as possible.

No sudden movements, please; you can throw your back out if you haven't done this type of stretching in a while. Reach to the point of gentle tension, never to the point of pain. Reach as far as you can at least three times, but do not bounce or "bob" forward with each reach.

Men's rankings	Age 40–49	Age 50–59	Age 60–69
Very fit	17 inches or more	16 inches or more	15 inches or more
Average	11–16 inches	10–15 inches	9–14 inches
Out of shape	8–10 inches	7–9 inches	6–8 inches
Couch potato	7 inches or less	6 inches or less	5 inches or less

Women's rankings	Age 40–49	Age 50–59	Age 60–69
Very fit	20 inches or more	19 inches or more	18 inches or more
Average	14–19 inches	13–18 inches	12–17 inches
Out of shape	11–13 inches	10– 12 inches	9–11 inches
Couch potato	10 inches or less	9 inches or less	8 inches or less

BETSY'S RACKET

Sowing exercise has reaped benefits for me

Just before writing this book I underwent a comprehensive physical exam, my first in a half-dozen years, at the Mayo Clinic satellite office in Jacksonville, Florida. At my age — 43 — I figured I was due.

After I gave urine and blood samples and was examined by Dr. Christian Van Den Berg, it was time for the infamous treadmill test. I was dressed in a blue sweatshirt (with just a sports bra underneath), blue corduroy pants, and well-worn tennis shoes. But when my name was called, a female technician named Jamie asked me to put on a hospital gown — one that opened in the front. Another female technician, Nancy, asked me to lie down. She opened up my gown and stuck at least eight electrodes to my chest, heart, and stomach area. They were *cold*.

"What are we trying to accomplish?" I asked Nancy after stepping on the fancy-looking treadmill.

"What this test does is show us how much your blood pressure elevates, how much your heart reacts under greater and greater stress, and how much oxygen intake your blood requires while under stress. If any `blips' show, that tells us that your heart does have a problem," Nancy explained.

"Normally, we start people off with 1.7 mph and a 10 percent incline for three minutes," she continued, "but we're going to skip that. I've set the machine to start at 2.5 mph and a 12 percent incline."

"Then what happens?" I inquired.

"Every three minutes, I will increase the speed by about 0.8 mph with a 12 percent increase in the treadmill's incline," Nancy said.

"Is there a finishing point to the test?"

"Yes," Nancy said. "The goal for you is completing an 18-minute test with the speed and incline increasing every three minutes."

The treadmill began moving slowly, and I walked steadily. This was no sweat — literally. After the first three minutes, the machine increased its load by roughly 12 percent; I was walking at a steady clip of 3.4 mph on a 14 percent incline. I walked briskly.

After six minutes of striding, I was barely breathing hard. My blood pressure had hardly moved. I was a little apprehensive about what was to come. The treadmill speed increased to 4.2 mph with an incline of 16 percent. I was still walking. At the nine-minute mark, technicians increased the treadmill speed to 5 mph with an 18 percent incline. Now I had to decide whether to walk really fast or break into a jog. I chose to keep walking, but at a very fast pace.

My forehead began glistening in sweat. Then the treadmill tilted up more and increased its speed at the 12-minute mark. I had to run when the machine increased to 5.5 mph and a 20 percent incline. I began sweating like a flop horse as rivulets of perspiration ran down my face. My soaking-wet pants were threatening to fall to my knees, as was a monitoring box strapped around my waist. I wanted a towel, a pair of running shorts, and a water jug.

I concentrated while the treadmill "ramped up" to its final setting at the 15-minute mark: 6.0 mph and a 22 percent incline. Since very few highways have an incline greater than 7 percent, I felt as though I was running up a tree! Still, I kept chugging away, determined to finish.

Finally, at the 18-minute mark, the treadmill stopped. The technician took my blood pressure for the eighth time while I wiped my sweat-soaked face with a towel. I had worked up a good lather, but it felt good to push my body. As I toweled off, I could see that Nancy and Jamie were happy with my results. My electrocardiogram lines were excellent — no blips.

"This clinic has been open 14 years," Jamie said, "and never in our history has any woman at any age been able to finish the test."

"You're kidding. You mean what I just finished?" I asked.

"Yes, I'm dead serious. Only two *men* of any age — one of them was an astronaut down at Cape Canaveral, I believe — have completed this test. What you have done is just amazing. Absolutely amazing. You are 233 percent above normal in functional aerobic capacity for someone your age. Most 43-year-old women can do this test for only nine minutes."

I was shocked, but the more I thought about it, my performance at the Mayo Clinic was the result of a 25-year commitment to getting in shape and *staying* in shape for the long haul. I had made that commitment early in my professional tennis career and stuck with it.

And then it hit me: *You reap what you sow.* If you sow exercise and fitness into your life, you will reap the benefits of good health and longevity.

Take a cold, hard look at the results. If you score well, treat yourself to a banana split (just kidding). If you're out of shape, that's okay, too. Increasing your regular physical activity by even a modest amount results in measurable long-term benefits.

Measuring the Shape You're In

The exercises in the last section measure how fit you are, more or less. You will find it useful to record where you stand on the fitness scale because you can use these statistics to gauge how much your fitness improves. Keep these results around so you can refer back to them in three to six months. If you make a steady, consistent attempt to get back in shape, you'll be glad that you have these measurements to refer back to.

You need to establish some other benchmarks, however. The following measurements relate to your weight and type of body frame. These will help you determine how successful you are in reducing the amount of fat you carry on your body.

Understanding your BMI

One fitness-scale method that you may hear more about these days is called the *Body Mass Index,* or BMI. Physicians and researchers who study obesity find the BMI to be their measurement of choice. BMI uses a mathematical formula that takes into account a person's height and weight. As a strict formula, the Body Mass Index equals a person's weight in kilograms divided by height in meters-squared. For those of you keeping score at home, that's $BMI = km/m^2$.

You may say to yourself: "I haven't done any equations since tenth-grade trigonometry, and besides, I don't know my weight and height in the Euro form of measurements."

Have no fear. I provide a converted Body Mass Index chart using inches and pounds. (See Table 3-1.) Just find your height in the left-hand column and run your finger across the columns over to your weight. The row above your weight (a number between 19 and 40) is your BMI.

For example, I stand 68 inches tall (that's 5 feet, 8 inches) and weigh 133 pounds. My finger finds number 68 in the left-hand column, slides over to the 131 and 138 boxes, and those boxes tell me I have a BMI of, oh, around 20.3.

Table 3-1

BMI Chart

Height in Inches	19	20	21	22	23	24	25	26	27	28	29	30	31	32	33	34	35	36	37	38	39	40
																			Weight in Pounds			
58	91	96	100	105	110	115	119	124	129	134	138	143	148	153	158	162	167	172	177	181	186	191
59	94	99	104	109	114	119	124	128	133	138	143	148	153	158	163	168	173	178	183	188	193	198
60	97	102	107	112	118	123	128	133	138	143	148	153	158	163	168	174	179	184	189	194	199	204
61	100	106	111	116	122	127	132	137	143	148	153	158	164	169	174	180	185	190	195	201	206	211
62	104	109	115	120	126	131	136	142	147	153	158	164	169	175	180	186	191	196	202	207	213	218
63	107	113	118	124	130	135	141	146	152	158	163	169	175	180	186	191	197	203	208	214	220	225
64	110	116	122	128	134	140	145	151	157	163	169	174	180	186	192	197	204	209	215	221	227	232
65	114	120	126	132	138	144	150	156	162	168	174	180	186	192	198	204	210	216	222	228	234	240
66	118	124	130	136	142	148	155	161	167	173	179	186	192	198	204	210	216	223	229	235	241	247
67	121	127	134	140	146	153	159	166	172	178	185	191	198	204	211	217	223	230	236	242	249	255
68	125	131	138	144	151	158	164	171	177	184	190	197	203	210	216	223	230	236	243	249	256	262
69	128	135	142	149	155	162	169	176	182	189	196	203	209	216	223	230	236	243	250	257	263	270
70	132	139	146	153	160	167	174	181	188	195	202	209	216	222	229	236	243	250	257	264	271	278
71	136	143	150	157	165	172	179	186	193	200	208	215	222	229	236	243	250	257	265	272	279	286
72	140	147	154	162	169	177	184	191	199	206	213	221	228	235	242	250	257	265	272	279	287	294
73	144	151	159	166	174	182	189	197	204	212	219	227	235	242	250	257	265	272	280	288	295	302
74	148	155	163	171	179	186	194	202	210	218	225	233	241	249	256	264	272	280	287	295	303	311
75	152	160	168	176	184	192	200	208	216	224	232	240	248	256	264	272	279	287	295	303	311	319
76	156	164	172	180	189	197	205	213	221	230	238	246	254	263	271	279	287	295	304	312	320	328

BMI, waistlines, and risk of disease

The accompanying chart describes your health risk based upon your BMI. The magic figure to watch out for is a BMI of 27 or 28, where doctors say they see more risk of diabetes, cardio-vascular problems, arthritis, certain cancers, and premature death. This is where you need to lose 10 or 15 pounds pronto to get your BMI under 25.

BMI	Weight Status	Waist Size	Health Risk
		Men: 40 or less	Men: Over 40
		Women: 35 or less	Women: Over 35
18.5 or less	Underweight	n/a	n/a
18.5 to 24.9	Normal	n/a	n/a
25.0 to 29.9	Overweight	Increased	High
30.0 to 34.9	Obese	High	Very high
35.0 to 39.9	Obese	Very high	Very high

If you like to play around on the Internet, type Body Mass Index into your search engine and find thousands of sites that calculate your BMI. You plug in two pieces of information: your height and your weight (in inches and pounds, no less!). You can also go straight to the Web address: www.consumer.gov/weightloss/bmi.htm.

What do the results mean? The higher your BMI, the higher your health risk. The risk increases even more if your waist size is greater than 40 inches for men or 35 inches for women.

I hate to use the "O" word because nobody likes to be called obese, but if your BMI places you in the obese category, you are packing too many pounds. (Obesity begins at 25 percent body fat for men and 30 percent for women.) Obesity contributes to cardiovascular and coronary heart disease, high cholesterol, high blood pressure, diabetes, and certain cancers.

Nearly 54 percent of American adults report being overweight, according to a 1998 survey by the Centers for Disease Control and Prevention. The CDC considers you overweight if you are up to 30 pounds over the target weight for your body frame size (see Tables 3-4 and 3-5). If you are 30 pounds or more above your target weight, the CDC says you are obese.

Determining your body frame size

Weight charts often ask for a body frame size so your ideal weight can be determined. The simplest — but least accurate — method to determine your frame size is to hold one of your wrists and try to touch your thumb and index finger. If your fingers do not touch, you're a big-boned person with a large body frame. If your thumb and index finger just meet, you have a medium frame. If they overlap, you have a small frame.

The more scientific approach involves calculating the ratio of your height in inches to the circumference of your wrist measured in inches. Yes, I know that sounds complicated. The wrist measurement should be taken closest to where your wrist meets your hand. Divide your height by the wrist measurement. Check Table 3-2 (for women) or Table 3-3 (for men) to see what your frame size is.

Table 3-2	Women's Height-to-Wrist Ratio
Inches	*Frame Sizes*
11 or higher	small
10.1 to 10.9	medium
10 or lower	large

Table 3-3	Men's Height-to-Wrist Ratio
Inches	*Frame Sizes*
10.4 or higher	small
9.6 to 10.3	medium
9.5 or lower	large

Weighing in

Now that you know your body frame size, you can calculate your ideal weight using Tables 3-4 and 3-5 from the Metropolitan Life Insurance Company:

Table 3-4		Ideal Weight Table for Men		
Feet	*Inches*	*Small*	*Medium*	*Large*
5	2	128–134	131–141	138–150
5	3	130–136	133–143	140–153
5	4	132–138	135–145	142–156
5	5	134–140	137–148	144–160
5	6	136–142	139–151	146–164
5	7	138–145	142–154	149–168
5	8	140–148	145–157	152–172
5	9	142–151	148–160	155–176
5	10	144–154	151–163	158–180
5	11	146–157	154–166	161–184
6	0	149–160	157–170	164–188
6	1	152–164	160–174	168–192
6	2	155–168	164–178	172–197
6	3	158–172	167–182	176–202
6	4	162–176	171–187	181–207

Table 3-5		Ideal Weight Table for Women		
Feet	*Inches*	*Small*	*Medium*	*Large*
4	10	102–111	109–121	118–131
4	11	103–113	111–123	120–134
5	0	104–115	113–126	122–137
5	1	106–118	115–129	125–140
5	2	108–121	118–132	128–143
5	3	111–124	121–135	131–147
5	4	114–127	124–138	134–151

Feet	Inches	Small	Medium	Large
5	5	117–130	127–141	137–155
5	6	120–133	130–144	140–159
5	7	123–136	133–147	143–163
5	8	126–139	136–150	146–167
5	9	129–142	139–153	149–170
5	10	132–145	142–156	152–173
5	11	135–148	145–159	155–176
6	0	138–151	148–162	158–179

Measuring your body fat in a pinch

You may want to know how much body fat your torso contains. My body fat ratio was important to me when I was playing professionally on the Women's Tennis Association tour, and I'm certainly more aware of the implications these days. Extra fat translates into extra weight, which causes your heart to work harder. At the same time, you need *some* fat on your body. Fat provides body insulation and protects the internal body organs. The body draws on fat when food intakes are low.

Most fitness clubs have plastic calipers or measuring instruments that give a snapshot measurement of body fat by pinching the skin on your midriff. The skinfold calipers are not highly accurate, but they are still worthwhile as a benchmark or starting point. You can use the calipers to measure your body fat on several areas of the body:

- ✔ Triceps (back of the upper arm)
- ✔ Chest (between the arm line and nipple)
- ✔ Subscapula (below the edge of the shoulder blade on the back)
- ✔ Waist (slightly to the right of the navel)
- ✔ Suprailium (over the hip bone)
- ✔ Thigh (halfway between the hip and knee joints)

Take at least two measurements at each site to ensure an accurate reading. Using this reading (your body-fat percentage), you can see how your body measures up to the average for your sex and age (see Figure 3-1).

Step on it!

The latest bathroom scale technology gives your weight *and* your body-fat percentage. When you step on the scale (your feet must be bare), the machine sends an imperceptible electric current through the body to measure differences in electrical resistance. Lean body tissue conducts electricity better than fatty tissue.

These body-fat bathroom scales are not perfect, but they are good enough to help you measure decreases in your body fat as you follow an exercise and weight-reduction program. (The price for these newfangled scales — between $80 and $150.)

Reviewing your stats

With your BMI, body frame size, and body fat results in hand, you should review the numbers like a Fortune 500 accountant inspects the company's quarterly profit-and-loss statement. Don't go off the deep end if you are heavier than you should be for your height. Let the results motivate you to improve your fitness level.

Your next step requires scheduling a physical with your family doctor. Be sure to arrive at your appointment with your results in hand.

Get Thee to a Doctor

If you haven't been exercising regularly for years or your exercise is relegated to weekend-warrior status, it's important that you see a physician before beginning a fitness program.

The American Medical Association (AMA) suggests that you have a medical checkup every one to three years if you are over 40. If several years have passed since you've visited a doctor, now's the time to make that appointment. I don't care if you ran every 10K race in the state when you were in your twenties or thirties, you still need a physician's clearance if you haven't exercised regularly in several years. To skip a medical checkup after the age of 40 is foolhardy at best and deadly at worst.

Body Fat Interpretation Chart
(as a percentage of total body weight)

Body fat percent - males

Age in Years															
Up to 20	6.2	8.5	10.5	12.5	14.3	16.0	17.5	18.9	20.2	21.3	22.3	23.1	23.8	24.3	24.9
21-25	7.3	9.5	11.6	13.6	15.4	17.0	18.6	20.0	21.2	22.3	23.3	24.2	24.9	25.4	25.8
26-30	8.4	10.6	12.7	14.6	16.4	18.1	19.6	21.0	22.3	23.4	24.4	25.2	25.9	26.5	26.9
31-35	9.4	11.7	13.7	15.7	17.5	19.2	20.7	22.1	23.4	24.5	25.5	26.3	27.0	27.5	28.0
36-40	10.5	12.7	14.8	16.8	18.6	20.2	21.8	23.2	24.4	25.6	26.5	27.4	28.1	28.6	29.0
41-45	11.5	13.8	15.9	17.8	19.6	21.3	22.8	24.7	25.5	26.6	27.6	28.4	29.1	29.7	30.1
46-50	12.6	14.8	16.9	18.9	20.7	22.4	23.9	25.3	26.6	27.7	28.7	29.5	30.2	30.7	31.2
51-55	13.7	15.9	18.0	20.0	21.8	23.4	25.0	26.4	27.6	28.7	29.7	30.6	31.2	31.8	32.2
56 & up	14.7	17.0	19.1	21.0	22.8	24.5	26.0	27.4	28.7	29.8	30.8	31.6	32.3	32.9	33.3

Body fat percent - females

Age in Years															
Up to 20	15.7	17.7	19.7	21.5	23.2	24.8	26.3	27.7	29.0	30.2	31.3	32.3	33.1	33.9	34.6
21-25	16.3	18.4	20.3	22.1	23.8	25.5	27.0	28.4	29.6	30.8	31.9	32.9	33.8	34.5	35.2
26-30	16.9	19.0	20.9	22.7	24.5	26.1	27.6	29.0	30.3	31.5	32.5	33.5	34.4	35.2	35.8
31-35	17.6	19.6	21.5	23.4	25.1	26.7	28.2	29.6	30.9	32.1	33.2	34.1	35.0	35.8	36.4
36-40	18.2	20.2	22.2	24.0	25.7	27.3	28.8	30.2	31.5	32.7	33.8	34.8	35.6	36.4	37.0
41-45	18.8	20.8	22.8	24.6	26.3	27.9	29.4	30.8	32.1	33.3	34.4	35.4	36.3	37.0	37.7
46-50	19.4	21.5	23.4	25.2	26.9	28.6	30.1	31.5	32.8	34.0	35.0	36.0	36.9	37.6	38.3
51-55	20.0	22.1	24.0	25.9	27.6	29.2	30.7	32.1	33.4	34.6	35.6	36.6	37.5	38.3	38.9
56 & up	20.7	22.7	24.6	26.5	28.2	29.8	31.3	32.7	34.0	35.2	36.3	37.2	38.1	38.9	39.5

Lean	Ideal	Average	Overfat

Figure 3-1:
Use this chart to see how your body-fat percentage measures up.

Expect your doctor to register some concern if

- You smoke cigarettes or puff on cigars.
- You are overweight by 20 or more pounds.
- You have a history of heart disease in your family.
- You receive an abnormal stress electrocardiogram (EKG) test.
- You complain about arthritis in your joints or bones.
- You have suffered from a debilitating illness in the last five years.

During a routine physical, your physician will check your eyes, ears, nose, throat, heart, weight, blood pressure, abdomen, lungs, neurological and skeletal systems, and urinary tract. Your height is measured to determine if osteoporosis has reduced your stature.

Screening for serious health conditions

As much as we may not want to admit it, health screenings in the forties and beyond can do more than just give us an assessment of where we measure up on the physical fitness scale. A routine exam is also a preventive measure that can save your life — or add many more quality years to your lifespan. Medical checkups enable you to discover serious health conditions, and catching a life-threatening disease early allows today's technological advances in medicine to work for you in ways that were not possible just ten or 20 years ago.

Cancer, which claims more than 500,000 lives each year, is the second most-common killer around (cardiovascular disease is first). The good news is that the rate of cancer deaths declined for the first time ever during the 1990s, thanks to early detection measures and fewer people smoking. During a medical exam, doctors usually look for signs of the following cancers:

Breast and cervical cancers

Women can expect an examination of their breasts and cervix and a Pap smear that may detect cervical cancer. Mammograms (breast X-rays) are indispensable in early detection of breast cancer; studies indicate that you are one-third less likely to develop breast cancer if you have regular mammograms. One in eight American women will develop breast cancer, and it's the leading cause of cancer death among women age 40 to 55.

Less common but no less serious is cervical cancer, which strikes a woman's reproductive tract and often results in invasive surgery to remove the uterus (hysterectomy). Radiation and chemotherapy are other forms of prevalent treatment. The overall five-year survival rate is 70 percent — and higher if caught early.

Colorectal cancer

A different type of cancer screening is recommended for individuals 50 and older: a test for colorectal cancer. Colon and rectal cancer develop in the digestive tract, which is also called the gastrointestinal (or GI) tract. Clinicians study the health of the rectum and colon with a viewing tube called an *endoscope*. No doubt about it, being "plumbed" by a lighted-viewing tube isn't something I'm looking forward to. But if I had cancer down there, I would want it detected as early as possible.

Prostate cancer

If you are a male, your physician should check your prostate at this time. The *prostate* — a walnut-sized gland located in the front of the rectum and just below the bladder — produces fluid for semen and has a tendency to enlarge in the middle-age years.

A prostate exam is a comeuppance time for guys, who get to drop their drawers, bend over, place their elbows on the examination table, and relax while a physician probes their rectums with a gloved finger. Don't feel too bad, fellows. Women have had to endure the discomforting pelvic exams since high school, so I think you'll survive a prostate exam. While unpleasant, the exam's over in a New York minute.

The doctor's highly trained index finger seeks information on the prostate's smoothness, tenderness, or any other abnormalities. The presence of nodules on the prostate may be a sign of prostate cancer, which is the most common non-skin cancer in American men these days. You're probably not aware that nearly as many men die from prostate cancer each year as women succumb to breast cancer.

Many high-profile men have faced prostate cancer. New York mayor Rudy Giuliani, General Norman Schwarzkopf, former U.S. Senator Bob Dole, New York Yankee manager Joe Torre, former junk-bond king Michael Milken, golfer Arnold Palmer, and singer Harry Belafonte have all been diagnosed with the disease. The good news is that the success rate of beating prostate cancer is excellent if caught early on.

Counting your heartbeats

When you inform your doctor that you intend to start an exercise program, he or she may suggest an EKG to look at any cardiovascular abnormalities. The *cardiovascular system* is the tree trunk of life, consisting of the heart, arteries, and veins. The heart contracts to force our blood — which contains life-essential oxygen and nutrients — to all of our body cells. Your doctor may look for signs of physical impairment in the cardiovascular system, because heart attacks kill and disable more people in the Western world than any other affliction.

An *EKG,* or electrocardiogram, is a reading of the electrical activity of your heart. Electrodes placed on the skin detect and graphically record your heart's electrical activity. An EKG is used in the diagnosis of heart disease.

Check out this checkup!

Following a medical checkup, Jerry Clark awaits the results.

"Mr. Clark," the doctor tells his anxious patient. "I'm afraid I have bad news. You only have six months to live."

Jerry sits in stunned silence for several minutes before regaining his composure. "I'm afraid I have no medical insurance," he says. "I can't possibly pay you in that time."

Replies the doctor, "Make that nine months."

 While smoking, obesity, and emotional stress are common causes of heart attacks, fairly strenuous physical activity significantly reduces those risks. If you want to live longer, exercising to raise your heartbeat is a great idea because 42 percent of all deaths are caused by cardiovascular disease. According to the American Heart Association, a lack of physical activity is a clear risk factor for heart disease. Get on that exercise bike!

Gauging your blood pressure

Nearly all health screenings start with a blood pressure test, but you can test yourself at a drugstore or supermarket pharmacy if you have a couple of quarters jangling in your pocket.

Your doctor won't overlook the results of a blood pressure test, and neither should you. High blood pressure, or *hypertension,* is an indicator that the force needed to push blood through your circulatory system is greater than normal. Most hypertension begins showing up before the age of 50.

In plain English, high blood pressure means your heart works too hard to pump blood through your arteries. It increases the risk of heart attacks, strokes, kidney failure, damage to the eyes, congestive heart failure, and atherosclerosis (a stage of hardening of the arteries involving fatty deposits inside the artery walls).

You hear two numbers when it comes to blood pressure readings, such as "You're 128 over 72," which is written 128/72. The top number refers to the *systolic pressure,* the reading when the heart is pumping; the lower number is the *diastolic pressure,* the reading between pumping actions. If you receive a systolic blood pressure of 140 or more and a diastolic reading of 90 or more, you are most likely suffering from hypertension.

If you have hypertension, your doctor will suggest several lifestyle changes — such as immediately starting an aerobic-based fitness program. Follow your doctor's orders and make the effort to perform regular cardiovascular exercise, which will lower your hypertension.

Because people with hypertension may not show any symptoms of a heart problem, they often go undiagnosed until complications occur. Regular blood pressure screenings can help your doctor diagnose and treat the problem and reduce the risk of further complications from hypertension.

Bend ze knees, please

Ask your doctor to examine your knees, because you'll be working them hard down the road, so to speak. The wear and tear on your knees from years of use may have produced slight tears in your knees' ligaments. Although the body usually tells you when the knees aren't 100 percent — through pain — you may have gotten used to a "bum" knee. You may have adjusted the way you walk and run to compensate. Knee problems are no fun. I've endured nine operations, and I could be due for another knee operation in the next year.

Doctors look at two ligaments of the knee that are most frequently injured — the *medial collateral ligament* and the *anterior cruciate ligament*. Medial collateral ligament injuries result from being struck on the lateral side of a firmly planted leg — a common injury in soccer, basketball, and football. If the force is sufficient, the anterior cruciate may also be damaged. A common cause of anterior cruciate tears is forced internal rotation of the knee — usually a sudden twist in the knee. Other causes of anterior cruciate ligament tears can occur in running or jumping sports. People who suffer such injuries often experience a tearing sensation or hear a "pop" — and it hurts! Some tears, however, are slight and hardly noticeable.

Don't be a hero. If the doctor asks, "Does the knee hurt when I twist it?" don't brush off the question. Your doctor must ask probing questions because he or she can do little more than feel around the knee and its ligaments. A skillful doctor may conduct certain tests by stretching your legs and knees into uncomfortable positions. Remember: Your feedback enables your doctor to make a proper diagnosis.

Don't think you have to baby your knees when you hit middle age. A Stanford University study tracked several hundred runners and nonrunners — ages 53 to 75 — for six years to find out if long-term running contributed to a corresponding increase in aches and pains. No correlation was found.

The remains of the exam

While your car is in the doctor's shop, he or she should look over the muscles and joints in your shoulders, ankles, and feet. In addition, a quick examination of your eyes is in order because your ability to see gradually diminishes with age.

The heart of the matter

You're not a spring chicken anymore. One of your concessions to age should be to regularly monitor your heart. The last time I checked, I counted only one onboard blood-pumping muscle, and this built-in computer sends out vital information regarding the health and welfare of your body.

You've probably forgotten your high school biology, but the following information is still true:

✔ Your heart is the strongest muscle in your body, beating an average of 100,000 beats daily or 4,166 times an hour. Your heart just beat four times in the time you took to read the previous sentence. If you live an average life span, you have 100 million heartbeats left!

✔ The heart has four chambers: two on the right and two on the left. As you exercise, blood returns to the right atrium depleted of oxygen and carrying carbon dioxide from the working muscles. The blood is then moved to the right ventricle, or pump, where the blood is pumped into the lungs to remove the carbon dioxide. Isn't this organ absolutely amazing? The blood, now brimming with oxygenated cells, collects in the left atrium before quickly moving to the left ventricle, where the heart pumps the enriched blood to the working body muscles.

✔ Your heart increases in size as you increase the time you exercise. If this fact surprises you, you've forgotten that the heart is a muscle just like any other defined muscles in your body.

The lenses of the eyes, after the age of 40, begin to thicken, decreasing your ability to focus on objects up close. This condition, known as *presbyopia,* cannot be reversed by exercise or medication. If your doctor detects presbyopia, he or she should refer you to an ophthalmologist for a complete eye examination.

Your doctor should also check your hearing. Men have more hearing problems than women and gradually lose the ability to hear high tones. If your doctor suspects significant hearing loss, he or she should refer you to a specialist who can prescribe hearing aids.

Chapter 4

The Lifetime Benefits of Being Physically Fit

• •

In This Chapter

▶ Creating physical margin

▶ Managing today's stress

▶ Enjoying a healthy sex life

▶ Feeling sexy in your senior years

• •

*T*here's a lot to like about being physically fit. I like the energy boost that a good workout gives me, the way my body stays trim, and the knowledge that exercise does a heart good. I like the way exercise gives me a sense of physical margin — a better chance to live longer and live better.

Let me explain this concept of physical margin further. Richard Swenson, M.D., an associate professor at the University of Wisconsin Medical School, authored a fascinating book several years ago called *Margin*. His basic hypothesis: When flying from New York's JFK Airport to Portland, Oregon, you need more than three minutes to change planes in Denver. More minutes are required to ensure you have time for problems that may occur during the changeover. This extra time you allow yourself to cover any possible snags in your travel plan is called a *margin*.

Just as you need to create time margin in your daily schedule, you must create *physical margin* — a buildup of stamina so that you can handle the upcoming middle-age years. You gain physical margin from the process of getting physically fit: doing 20 to 30 minutes of aerobic activity three or more times a week, along with muscle-strengthening and -stretching activities twice a week. (See Chapter 6 for more on these three aspects of fitness.)

The Benefits Are Hardly Marginal

With physical margin, you may attack life with a properly conditioned body that maintains energy reserves. These reserves may be called upon when you experience mental and physical stresses. Physical margin gives you the ability to battle illnesses and presents you with a better shot at living longer.

When you have become physically fit and created physical margin in your life, you:

- ✔ Reduce your risk of dying prematurely (especially from heart disease).
- ✔ Reduce your risk of developing high blood pressure.
- ✔ Reduce your risk of developing colon cancer.
- ✔ Reduce your feelings of depression and anxiety.
- ✔ Help control your weight.
- ✔ Help build and maintain healthy bones, muscles, and joints.
- ✔ Become stronger and better able to perform tasks.
- ✔ Promote your psychological well-being.

"Starting to exercise is comparable, from a health benefit standpoint, to quitting smoking," says Stanford University exercise and health researcher Ralph Paffenbarger Jr. His findings from a 1995 study, "Physical Activity and Cardiovascular Health," state:

- ✔ **Regular exercise lessens your chance of developing cardiovascular disease or high blood pressure**. In addition, regular exercise may lessen your risk of cancer, osteoporosis — and even the common cold. Your mental health improves as well; your regular exercise routine helps you control your stress, anxiety, sleep, and depression problems.

- ✔ **Vigorous exercise may extend your life.** Dr. Paffenbarger says, "All adults should set and reach a goal of accumulating at least 30 minutes of moderate-intensity physical activity on most, and preferably all, days of the week."

You invite overall good health to visit and stay with you a long time when you exercise regularly. Your mood will improve, and you'll feel better about yourself — developments that could even impact your relationships with close loved ones. Your partner will notice the spring in your step and your sunnier disposition.

You Can Cut the Stress with a Knife

More than 160 years ago, Alexis de Tocqueville, the French commentator on life in the young United States, observed that Americans were always in a hurry. Life in the States hasn't changed much, has it? And Americans are not the only folks hustling on the planet. Everyone seems to be walking at a more harried pace these days.

The advancements in technology, medicine, transportation, and telecommunications make your life pretty good, or do they? You may have *too* much stimulation coming your way, and that stimulation may cause stress. *Stress* may be defined as any condition or situation that requires a person to make physical and/or psychological adjustments. Here are some examples of different levels of stress:

✔ **Mild**

- Running late to the airport
- Not finding your car keys

✔ **Moderate**

- Working to make a project deadline
- Planning an extended holiday

✔ **Severe**

- Losing your job or uncertainty about your job's future
- Impending retirement
- Learning of a loved one or friend contracting a serious illness

Exercise is an excellent antidote to stress. Here are some examples of how exercise may help reduce your daily stresses:

✔ Huffing and puffing on the treadmill, for example, blows off steam like a teakettle.

✔ Walking in the quiet of the morning helps you prepare for your day by giving you time to think about your schedule — what you need to accomplish, whom you need to call, and what appointments you must keep.

✔ An energetic tennis game during the work day stimulates the mind and provides a mental break from reading reports and crunching numbers.

✔ A low-intensity sport like golf provides a welcome change of scenery from the home or office.

> ✔ Exercising after work — instead of sitting in frustrating rush-hour traffic — may be a two-for-one way to reduce stress: (1) You exercise and (2) You drive when less traffic is on the road.
>
> ✔ Doing yard work or going on a spring cleaning binge may provide a quick-fix for your stress. You also feel some degree of accomplishment.

Although exercising adds another time commitment to your life, it doesn't seem to create *more* stress. David Nieman, an Appalachian State University researcher, put a control group of "stressed-out" women (as determined by psychological testing) on a brisk walking program. After a month of walking, he tested them against a sedentary control group and found that the walking women "maintained an elevated mood."

Increasing your capacity for tolerating physical stresses deepens your ability for tolerating *all* stresses. Theories abound regarding the different reasons why exercise improves your mental health and reduces stress. Researchers agree that cardiovascular exercise helps people feel better and function better under stress. Other researchers point to endorphins and other feel-good chemicals released by the body during exercise.

Sports psychologist Dr. Jim Loehr says that the release of these powerful chemicals (such as catecholamine, adrenaline, noradrenaline, hydrocortisone, and glucocorticoid) causes immune cells to flood the cardiovascular system, helping to protect the body against illness. I tend to think that fitness is a therapeutic time-out that builds self-confidence and helps people ward off stress.

Perhaps you've lived so long with stress that you don't even know what life would be like *without* it. You may not have many options for coping with a stressful situation (for example, the terminal illness of a spouse), but exercise is one of the few weapons you have for dealing with it. I firmly believe that exercising today can reduce stress tomorrow.

Being Fit Helps Your Sex Life

With a title like that, I have a feeling that you won't skip this section.

Everyone is interested in improving their sex lives. Sex enriches your life in a unique way. Making love is a form of "sexercise" — an athletic activity that has physical release. The act of love is good for the heart and muscles, reduces stress, and induces feelings of happiness and well-being. Well-established research confirms that the soft touch of physical intimacy, when coupled with emotional intimacy, is good for the body and soul. An active sex life may motivate couples to maintain their fitness levels — or lose those "love handles." If the physical relationship is important to you, being physically fit enhances your experience.

For those dealing with low libido, getting fit and losing weight may increase your sexual appetite. Sexual desire is set in the brain, which, in turn, is influenced by factors that include how you view your physical body, your energy level, and your health. You can do something about all three by exercising regularly. A fitness program tones your body, results in weight loss, boosts your energy level, and leaves you feeling healthy. These positive changes are going to result in a better sex life.

For those of you who say you are too tired for sex by the time lights are switched off, the answer is to get started on your exercise program! You may think that stair stepping three times a week or joining a tennis league makes you even *more* tired, but the opposite is true. Consistent exercise stimulates helpful enzymes in your muscles and cardiovascular system — you gain more energy to attack your day and still leave some fuel in the tank for bedtime.

For the men

Many men are unaware that their bodies and reproductive organs are undergoing subtle but unmistakable changes in their middle-age years. The reason is related to lessening amounts of testosterone. *Testosterone* is the male hormone largely responsible for sexual desire and the body's natural strength. As age and the decline in the level of testosterone set in, gradual changes occur that catch many men off guard.

Men in their forties can't help but notice a couple of things: (1) They aren't as strong as they used to be and (2) They are having difficulty getting erections as effortlessly as in the past. I have two names for the latter affliction: impotence or erectile dysfunction.

In case you didn't notice, erectile dysfunction is the new, improved, politically correct label for impotence. Perhaps you read those annoying "Improve Your Sex Life" ads displayed on the sports pages — the ones asking whether you have erection problems and promising "Separate waiting rooms to ensure your privacy. *All it takes is a toll-free call.*"

To tell the truth, 10 percent of the American male population is impotent by the age of 50; by age 60, that percentage climbs to nearly 20. Impotence affects some 30 million American men, but only 10 percent seek medical help, further underscoring the shame males feel when this affliction affects them.

Exercise is very important to your sexual health. Working out isn't going to cure impotence, but a steady, consistent exercise program that raises your heart rate at least three times a week pushes more blood throughout the body's veins and arteries. A strong heart increases blood flow and circulation in your reproductive area, and that increased blood flow helps you remain virile and effective under the bed sheets.

So the next time you decide whether or not to step on that treadmill, remind yourself that vigorous exercise does a lot more than improve cardiovascular fitness. That thought should get your feet running.

For the women

Say you're a woman in your forties. You always experience regular menstrual periods, but you miss a period or two. When you do menstruate, your flow is notably different from before. You never had trouble sleeping before, but two or three nights a week you can't sleep. Oh, one other occurrence: Your sex life is different. You find making love more difficult because your vagina doesn't lubricate as it did before. These symptoms are all part of being perimenopausal. (See Chapter 2 for more on perimenopause.). The decreasing amounts of estrogen released into your body during your cycle affect nearly every organ in your body. And it can get to your head, too: You may think that menopause may signal the end of your days as an attractive, desirable, and sexual woman.

Exercise helps you deal with these issues. When you get physically fit, trim some pounds, and sport a sunny complexion, you feel self-confident, attractive, and sexually desirable to your spouse or partner. When you feel sexually desirable, your self-esteem lifts. Exercise helps you feel good about yourself, which helps you feel more "sexy." The person you love the most appreciates your attitude and your desire to "not let yourself go."

Whether you're perimenopausal or menopausal, physical fitness gives your body an opportunity to release pent-up tension while allowing the brain to produce endorphins that relieve any aches and pains. Just as exercise is recommended to relieve some of your daily stresses (including premenstrual syndrome), physical activity energizes you in your pre- and post-menopausal years.

Burning a Slow and Steady Fire: Sex in Your Senior Years

Today's sexual relationship is an investment in your future sexual relationship. When you pass this middle-age scene, two of the things that give you your greatest joys — your children and career — may no longer take up as much time as they once did. This extra time means that your relationship with your loved one steps up in importance. Perhaps you know couples in their senior years whose happiness and devotion to each other may be seen on their faces. These couples are the ones still walking arm-in-arm with a gleam in their eyes that announces to the whole world that their love is intimate and lifelong. With maturity, you too may recognize that sex expresses joy and affirms life.

My research indicates that although the frequency of sex may be reduced by advancing age, the meaning of the sexual relationship may be deepened. The intimacy an older couple shares may be more enriching and satisfying with the passage of years. Yet many people, as they grow older, poke fun at their diminishing abilities to perform sexually. The following joke is one of my favorites.

The following are the three stages of a couple's love life:

1. Couples in their twenties have sex triweekly.

2. Couples in their thirties try weekly to have sex.

3. Couples in their forties, fifties, and sixties *try weakly* to have sexual relations.

Sex begins upstairs — in the mind. When you *think* you're too old or too tired for sex, you *act* accordingly. This way of thinking is a shame because couples can — and should — enjoy a vibrant sex life until they are well into their seventies, even their eighties. Affection, warmth, and sensuality do not have to deteriorate with age as long as we stay in good physical shape. If you don't want to *try weakly* to have sexual relations, now's the time to get back into the gym. Then you'll truly enjoy a love for a lifetime.

Chapter 5

Eating for Fitness and Health

. . . .

In This Chapter

▶ Adopting healthy eating habits

▶ Cutting down on fat

▶ Following the Ten Commandments of Good Nutrition

▶ Drinking more water to ensure good health

. . . .

*O*ne of life's joys is eating food; in fact, 84 percent of Americans named eating as their top leisure-time activity in a Harris survey. Instead of eating to live, however, you live to eat. You snack on tortilla chips and guacamole dip all afternoon long while State U battles its arch rivals on the gridiron, you fire up the barbecue and prepare mountains of food as a way of showing affection for friends and family, and you conduct business while indulging in savory entrees prepared for you in restaurants and bistros.

People all over the world — but particularly in North America — love food high in fat, low in fiber, and rich in chocolate. No wonder why too many of us are losing the Battle of the Bulge — and becoming more and more unmotivated to do anything about it.

But if you want to get fit or stay fit after 40, then *what* you eat, *when* you eat, and *how much* you eat become critical. It's not going to do your body good to start a thrice-weekly workout program at the local gym if you don't bring a corresponding discipline to the dinner table. Eating healthy will help you lose weight quicker, get you into better shape sooner, and give you a greater opportunity to travel through life feeling better.

Words to Live By: Eat Less, Exercise More

If one of the reasons you're reading *Fit Over 40 For Dummies* is to shed some pounds while you get back into shape, there is one boring, unchangeable truth that you should know: If you want to lose weight, you should eat less and exercise more. Do the math. A pound of fat equals approximately 3,500 calories. If you eat 500 fewer calories a day, you can lose one pound in one week. If you exercise away another 500 calories a day, you can lose two pounds in a week.

If you're going to invest time and effort to improve your body — and if you're reading these words, there's a good chance you are — you might as well get the best return on that investment. That translates into eating smarter and eating less. No, the latter advice does not mean you should subject yourself to starvation-level diets; essential nutrients are hard to come by in diets of less than 2,000 calories a day.

Eat less and live longer?

When Dr. Roy Walford was a UCLA research scientist in the pathology department, he conducted experiments in which laboratory mice were given less and less to eat — but always enough to live on. To Dr. Walford's surprise, the deprived mice lived longer than their well-fed counterparts.

Dr. Walford wondered if the same theory held true for humans. Offering himself as a human lab experiment for the last 20 years, the research scientist has voluntarily chosen to eat very little — a little over 1,600 calories a day — in an effort to live to 120 years of age. At the printing of this book, Dr. Walford is 75 years of age and in excellent health. Walford stands 5'8" and weighs just 134 pounds. He shaves his head and sports a long Fu Manchu moustache, which makes him look 10 to 20 years younger. His physique is excellent; Walford works out with weights every other day at a gym close to his Los Angeles home.

Walford's epiphany came when he noticed that middle-aged mice live 20 percent longer when eased into a restricted-calorie diet. His search for the fountain of youth has led to a dietary regimen that consists of small servings of low-fat milk shakes, vegetable salads, fish, and baked sweet potatoes. His daily calorie count of 1,600 is about half the 3,000 calories per day that are consumed by most Americans.

Will a subsistence-level diet result in longer life? In Walford's case, he won't know for another 10, 20, or 30 years. The proof is in the pudding — low-fat, of course.

If you're trying to limit yourself to 2,000 calories a day, government dietary guidelines recommend that you get less than 30 percent of your daily calories from fat. What does this mean in practical terms? You should try to eat foods that average three grams of fat for every 100 calories. Deluxe fast-food hamburgers generally have 40 to 50 percent of their calories from fat, so you're going to have to balance that meal with something low-fat — like salad with no-fat dressing.

Most people know that good nutrition is essential to feeling our best and reaching our optimal fitness levels. How you get there could be the subject of a book. (Come to think of it, it *is* the subject of many books.) The point of this chapter is that overeating and eating the wrong foods can negate any gains made in the gym faster than you can say "I'll supersize that order." The best advice on nutrition as it relates to fitness is summed up in the next section.

The Ten Commandments of Nutrition

I've asked an acquaintance of mine — Pamela Smith, a nationally known nutritionist, author (*The Diet Trap* and *Eat Well, Live Well),* and culinary consultant from Orlando — how you can eat healthier and become fitter by doing so.

Eating well may be challenging, but it can be done, says Pam, and it's not as complicated as you think. Pam's "Ten Commandments of Great Nutrition" emphasize what you should eat, rather than what to avoid. Keep these commandments, and you won't wander 40 years in the fitness wilderness before reaching the Promised Land.

1: Thou shalt never skip breakfast

Your body awakens in a slowed-down state. When you don't eat breakfast to meet your body's demand for energy and boost the metabolic system, your body turns to its own muscle mass (not fat!) for energy. Your metabolism slows down even more, as your body conserves energy for a potentially long, starved state. Your next meal — lunch or dinner — is not burned for energy, but stored as fat. (Your body is trying to keep you from starving to death!) You need to give your body a chance to boost its energy and raise its metabolism by feeding it some breakfast daily.

II: Thou shalt eat every three to four hours and have a healthy snack handy

Once you begin your day with breakfast, your goal should be to keep your system working for you. To prevent your blood-sugar level from dropping and to keep your metabolic rate high, you need to digest your food at regular intervals throughout the day. Your blood-sugar level normally crests and falls every three to four hours. As your blood-sugar level begins to fall, so does your energy — along with your mood, your concentration, and your ability to handle stress.

Letting many hours pass between meals causes the body to slow down metabolically. When you allow too much time to pass between lunch and dinner, your dinner (healthy or not) is perceived as an overload; the nutrients are not being used optimally, and your lowered blood-sugar level leaves you sleepy and craving sweets. When you eat frequent, small meals, your body has a chance to metabolize those calories efficiently — burning those calories for energy instead of storing them as fat.

Several small meals a day deposit less fat than one or two large meals. You must keep your body fed with food at the right time to metabolize calories efficiently.

III: Thou shalt always eat a carbohydrate with a protein

Eating at regular intervals throughout the day is not the only important factor in keeping your metabolism running fast and your body working well. Every meal (and snack) should include both carbohydrates and proteins.

Carbohydrates — fruits, fruit juices, and non-starchy vegetables — provide 100 percent pure energy and fuel for your body to burn. *Proteins* — meats and dairy products — are essential for your skin, bones, ligaments, and cell growth among other complex functions. When no carbohydrates are available, the body burns proteins. Eat a carbohydrate with a protein to protect the protein from being wasted as a less efficient fuel source. Example: eating wild rice and salad (carbs) along with a baked, skinless chicken breast (protein).

You need protein for boosting your metabolism, building your body muscle, keeping your body fluids in balance, and healing and fighting infections. But protein is so potent that you don't need much of it. The Recommended Daily Allowance is 0.36 grams per pound of body weight (0.8 grams per kilogram), which translates into 63 grams of protein for males weighing 175 pounds and

50 grams for females weighing 140 pounds. This means a woman would receive the protein she needs by eating just six ounces of chicken. (Table 5-1 lists other sources of protein.)

IV: Thou shalt double thy fiber

Grandma used to say, "Eat your roughage." Now I counsel you to *double* your fiber. Increasing your fiber intake may be accomplished by eating wholesome foods prepared in a wholesome way:

- Eat whole grain breads and cereals instead of white, refined types. Look for "100 percent whole wheat" on the label with the word "whole" as the first ingredient on the list.
- Eat fresh vegetables and fruits with well-washed skins. Peel vegetables and fruits that have been waxed.

Table 5-1	Protein Sources	
Food	*Serving Size*	*Protein*
chicken (skinless)	4 ounces	35 g
cottage cheese (1 – 2%)	1 cup	28 g
cream cheese (nonfat)	1 ounce	4 g
egg (white)	1 large	3 g
fish (cod, salmon)	6 ounces	40 g
lamb (lean)	4 ounces	30 g
meat (lean, red)	4 ounces	35 g
milk (low or nonfat)	1 cup	8 g
pork (lean)	4 ounces	35 g
tofu (low-fat)	6 ounces	30 g
tuna (water-packed)	6 ounces	40 g
turkey (skinless)	4 ounces	35 g
yogurt (low-fat)	1 cup	13 g

- ✔ Choose rawer or lightly cooked vegetables in a nonprocessed form. (As vegetables are ground, mashed, pureed, or juiced, the fiber effectiveness decreases.)
- ✔ Add a variety of legumes (such as peas or beans) to your diet.
- ✔ Add unprocessed oat or wheat bran to your foods. Try eating bran as a hot cereal or by sprinkling it uncooked on your cold cereal.

V: Thou shalt trim the fat from thy diet

Fat is a nutrient that the body needs in very limited amounts for lubrication and for transporting fat-soluble vitamins (A, D, E, and K). When eaten in excess, fat

- ✔ Increases your cholesterol level and in turn your risk of heart disease and stroke.
- ✔ Increases your risk of developing cancer, particularly of the colon.
- ✔ Increases your risk of gall bladder disease.
- ✔ Elevates your blood pressure, regardless of your weight.
- ✔ Makes you fat!

People need to eat carbohydrates and proteins at each meal; they don't need fats in the quantities the average person consumes. One ounce of fat supplies twice the number of calories as one ounce of carbohydrate or protein. Research shows that fats from foods are stored as fat on the body more readily than carbohydrates or proteins. Fewer fats in your diet means less fat on your body and less cholesterol in your blood. (See "Reducing Your Fat Intake" in this chapter for more on fats.)

VI: Thou shalt believe thy mother was right: Eat thy vegetables

Vegetables and fruits are carbohydrates that provide a storehouse of vitamins, minerals, and other substances to protect against disease. Fruits and veggies are also valuable no-fat, no-cholesterol sources of fiber and fluid.

Generally the more vivid the fruit or vegetable's color, the more essential nutrients it holds. That deep orange or red coloring in carrots, sweet potatoes, cantaloupes, apricots, peaches, and strawberries signals their vitamin A content. Dark green leafy vegetables such as greens, spinach, romaine lettuce, Brussels sprouts, and broccoli are loaded with vitamin A as well as folic acid (a B vitamin that is essential for cell growth and reproduction). Vitamin C is found in more than just citrus fruits; it is also power-packed into strawberries, cantaloupes, tomatoes, green peppers, and broccoli. When veggies are loaded with color, they're loaded with nutrition!

VII: Thou shalt get thy vitamins and minerals from food, not pills

Can good nutrition be put into a capsule? No! Do you need to take vitamin-mineral supplements? It depends on your lifestyle choices.

Do you skip breakfast? Lunch too, sometimes? Do you eat on the run a lot? Eat out frequently? Drink alcohol? Have a high-stress career or home life? Drink coffee? If you answer yes to a few of these questions, your nutritional state may be at risk. If you continue this lifestyle, you may benefit from supplemental vitamins and minerals. However, supplements may not be the answer to repairing your nutritional imbalance. You may remedy your situation by arranging your day to include eating balanced, wholesome meals and snacks at regular intervals. Just figure out *what* to grab and *when* to grab it.

VIII: Thou shalt drink at least eight glasses of water a day

Increasing your water intake to meet your body's needs may produce miraculous results. Water reduces fat deposits in the body, flushes out waste and toxins, helps maintain muscle tone, moisturizes skin, and even suppresses appetite. (You can chug-a-lug much more information about the benefits of water in Chapter 19).

Water makes up 92 percent of your blood plasma, 80 percent of your muscle mass, 60 percent of your red blood cells, and 50 percent of everything else in your body. What an important ingredient to your body's makeup!

How much water do you need? Eight to ten glasses each day. As you begin to meet this need by drinking more water, your natural thirst for it increases. As you figure out what water does for your body, your motivation for drinking it grows. Drinking water is habit-forming — the more you drink, the more you want.

IX: Thou shalt consume minimum amounts of sugar, salt, caffeine, and alcohol

Called by many names — honey, brown sugar, corn syrup, fructose — sugar is sugar. Sugar causes dental cavities, obesity, and mood swings; it wreaks havoc with diabetes and hypoglycemia. Cut back on your daily use of sugar and eat more fruit to satisfy your natural craving for a sweet taste. Sugar abuse is not worth robbing yourself of precious energy and stamina.

As for salt, most people consume five to 25 times more than they need, leading to hypertension and kidney disease. Caffeine, a relatively mild stimulant, promotes irritability, anxiety, and mood disturbances. As for alcohol, one of the most common and addictive drugs of our time, much medical research is implicating excess alcohol as a factor in many killer diseases: hypoglycemia (abnormally low blood sugar), brain and heart damage, enlarged blood vessels in the skin, chronic gastritis, and pancreatitis (inflammation of the pancreas).

X: Thou shalt never go on a fad diet

Why is weight so easy to gain and so hard to lose? Why is extra weight so hard to keep off? The solution begins with an acknowledgement: Weight is not the problem, weight is only the symptom. Your eating patterns and perspectives about food are the problems. You may eat, not to meet your body's physical needs for nourishment, but for other reasons, often emotionally based. Freedom from weight issues comes only from dealing with the problems, not the symptom.

The word "diet" can be a nasty four-letter word. Diet speaks defeat and depression and denotes temporary action. You may go on diets only to go off them. Diets don't work; they modify behavior only temporarily.

Break the diet mentality with a nutrition consciousness that works for life. You can feel better, have abundant energy from morning to night, and look more radiant and healthy. You need to take a second look at your eating habits; with your newfound knowledge about nutrition and the way your body works, you should never have to diet again!

Reducing Your Fat Intake

Physicians Robert Buxbaum and Lyle Micheli, authors of *Sports for Life,* say that the average American's calorie consumption has *decreased* slightly since

1910, but average fat consumption has *risen* by 30 percent. Fat, while useful as an energy reserve, is stored when not needed — and stored around the midsection. Every time you enjoy a lip-smacking bacon-double-cheeseburger-deluxe-with-gobs-of-secret-sauce, you are swallowing more than 60 grams of artery-clogging fat — a little less than the daily recommended amount. Add a bag of fries, and caution lights should be going off in your head.

Like any worthwhile goal, reducing your personal fat intake requires some effort and commitment. Figuring out how to bring the flavor out of food without adding fat, order more healthy meals at restaurants, and discover nutritious snack foods is not easy. But the benefits far exceed the effort. To get you started, here are some ideas from Pam Smith to trim the fat when grocery shopping:

- ✔ **Switch from whole-milk dairy products to skim or 1 percent milk and nonfat plain yogurt.** Look for fat-free or lower-fat versions of your favorite cheeses. Ricotta, mozzarella, cottage, and cream cheese all come in low-fat versions. Check the label to be sure these dairy products have fewer than 5 grams of fat per ounce.

- ✔ **At the deli, go for the leanest meats.** Select sliced turkey, chicken, or lean ham. Limit your use of high-fat, high-sodium sausages and processed meats, such as hot dogs, bacon, and salami.

- ✔ **Buy whole-grain and freshly baked breads and rolls.** Whole-grain baked goods have more natural flavor and do not need the addition of butter or margarine to taste good.

- ✔ **Use the new all-fruit jams on breads or toast.** Rather than spreading on the fat with butter or margarine, you can enjoy your morning toast with a naturally sweet jam.

- ✔ **Keep an abundant supply of fresh fruits and precut munchy vegetables on hand for snacking.** Buy light popcorn and low-fat crackers rather than chips and cookies. Substitute sorbet or frozen juice bars for ice cream. Nonfat frozen yogurts may also be consumed sparingly; although nonfat frozen yogurt contains no fat, it is higher in sugar than most ice cream.

- ✔ **When you're dining out, order any sauces, dressings, toppings, or spreads on the side.** You control the portions. The typical restaurant meal contains the fat equivalent of 12 to 14 pats of butter.

- ✔ **Watch those portions when you are dining out.** Most restaurants serve twice as much food as you need. Order "lite eaters" portions or take leftovers home for a great meal tomorrow.

Restricting your calories in one move

Looking for a great exercise that's guaranteed to keep your weight under control? Let me teach you how to perform the "push-out" at the dining table. In this exercise, you place the palms of your hands against the table and slowly push you and your chair away from the table. Feel the slow burn in your arms. This non-aerobic exercise isolates the triceps and biceps and is quite effective in reducing body fat and shedding

unwanted pounds. This powerful movement must be practiced consistently to have any long-term effect.

I'm being facetious, of course, but the "push-out" may become the most effective exercise in your new program. So, the next time you dine, remember to push out before you push more food into your mouth!

Overcoming the Desire to Overeat

Overeating is a problem for many people trying to lose weight. Although most excess body fat is caused more often by decreased physical activity than anything else, the truth is, you probably still eat too much, too often. Here are some tips to prevent overeating:

- ✔ **Have a few sips of orange juice before you eat.** Several ounces of juice will raise your blood sugar and take the edge off your hunger pains.

- ✔ **Eat with company.** When you're eating alone and have no one to talk to, you're liable to keep eating and eating, because food is your friend. Wait until family members are home before serving dinner or try to eat with a friend. Polite dinner conversation may put the focus on family or friends and off the food.

- ✔ **Learn to live with smaller portions.** Where is it written that you have to cover every square inch of your plate with heaping helpings? The first couple of times you put less food on your plate, your body may demand more. Stick with the program — your body may get use to smaller portions. If you're the type who just can't say no to a second helping of a tasty main course (my weakness is lasagna), help yourself to a second helping of salad or vegetables instead.

- ✔ **Eat slower.** When you wolf down your food in three minutes, you may want to extend the eating experience by scavenging for second helpings.

- ✔ **Eat some fruit between meals.** Face it: You probably overeat because you wait until a regular mealtime to chow down. If you eat an orange or banana between lunch and dinner, it stands to reason that you may be less hungry when you sit down to the dinner table.

Eating less at lunch

You're not doing yourself much good when you eat like a glutton at lunchtime and eat less at dinner. Here are some midday tactics you may want to adopt:

✔ **Pack less in your lunch.** Maybe you pack two big halves of a sandwich into your lunch box because you've been packing your lunch this way since your first job out of college. A half sandwich should do just fine.

✔ **Ditch the chips.** Salty, artery-clogging chips may be replaced with raw carrots, dried fruit, or more healthy snacks.

✔ **Stay out of the company cafeteria and nearby restaurants.** Why tempt yourself with shrimp penne pasta or breaded chicken? Eat the lunch you bring from home.

✔ **Exercise during your lunch hour.** When you exercise before you eat, you're not as hungry.

✔ **Eat one dessert a day.** Listen, I'm the biggest chocoholic out there, but even I know that I can't have two or three desserts a day and expect to keep my weight down.

✔ **Drink plenty of water.** You're not going to be as hungry if you're drinking eight to ten glasses of water a day.

✔ **Use a fork and knife.** Even when you're eating take-out pizza, use a fork and knife. Using utensils slows you down and enables you to take smaller bites. Smaller bites means more chewing; more chewing enables you to savor your food longer; savoring your food longer means you may eat less.

Part II
Exploring Your Options

The 5th Wave   By Rich Tennant

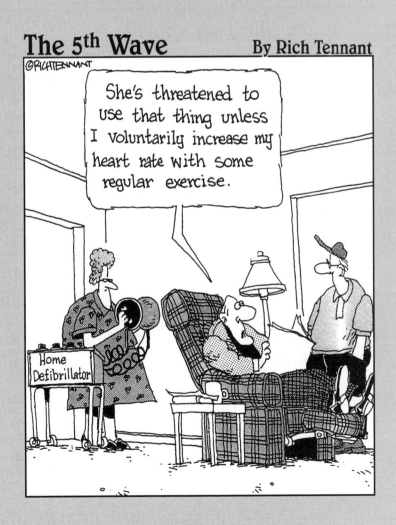

In this part . . .

Time to look over the fitness landscape and see what's out there. Chapter 6 explains the differences between the Big Three of fitness — aerobic, anaerobic, and stretching exercises — and why you need to incorporate all of them into a well-rounded fitness program. You'll learn how to monitor your heart rate to ensure that you're reaching the rate that is best for you.

This part also introduces you to the various types of exercise machinery you will encounter at a gym — or even in your den. You'll learn what each machine can do for you and why you really should do some weight training on strength machines. This part will also help you decide whether to work out in a fitness center, at work, or in your home.

Chapter 6

The Big Three: Aerobic, Anaerobic, and Stretching Exercises

*W*hen middle-aged people think about starting to exercise again, they generally see themselves walking on a treadmill or pedaling a stationary bike — and that's it. Although aerobic exercise is important — the foundation of your exercise regimen — it is only one of *three* types of exercise that you should do to shape, tone, and define your body. Combining all three will give you the most complete workout possible.

You should include these three forms of exercise in your regimen:

✔ **Aerobic:** The body is said to be working *aerobically* when it operates at a pace that allows the cardio-respiratory system (the lungs, heart, and bloodstream) to replenish energy as you exercise. Put another way, aerobic exercise causes the body to use oxygen to create energy. This is basically anything that gets the heart going, like walking on treadmills, cycling on stationary bikes, or stepping on stair stepper machines.

✔ **Anaerobic:** *Anaerobic* exercise causes the body to make energy without oxygen because the demand for energy is so fast and huge that the body must create it from numerous natural body chemicals. Anaerobic exercise is any form of nonsustained physical activity that typically involves a limited number of specific muscles over a short time, such as strength training or lifting free weights.

> ✔ **Stretching:** Don't forget about this one. Stretching increases your range of motion and prevents muscle strain and injuries. Stretching helps your joints stay healthy, keeps circulation levels high, and allows you to recover more quickly from your workouts.

This chapter will tell you what you need to know about these three types of exercise and describe why *anaerobic* exercise is a must if you want to lose weight and get in shape.

The Heart of Fitness: Aerobic Exercise

The great thing about aerobic exercise is that you can mix 'n' match. You can embark on a Saturday afternoon hike in the mountains, golf on Sunday, walk on a treadmill on Tuesday, play tennis on Thursday, and use a stepper machine on Friday — and you'll be way ahead of the fitness curve. (See the sidebar "Is my activity aerobic?" for a list of activities that are usually considered aerobic.)

Entering the training zone

The American College of Sports Medicine recommends that aerobic activities be performed three to five times a week, for 20 to 60 minutes on each occasion. When performing aerobic exercise, you need to be aware of what the maximum heart rate and target heart rates are. For those of us over 40 years of age, our focal point should be reaching the "training zone" or target heart rate, which is the range between 60 percent and 80 percent of your maximum heart rate. Working within this zone gives you the maximum health and fat-burning benefits from your cardiovascular activity.

I could give you a complicated mathematical formula to figure out your target heart rate, but it's just easier to look at Figure 6-1 and eyeball what your target heart rate should be. For a more precise method, you could go to healthchecksystems.com and calculate your minimum and maximum training heart rates based on whether you are a intermediate, beginning, or advanced exerciser.

Monitoring your heart rate

Knowing how fast your heart beats while you stride on that treadmill or ride that bicycle is important. (And, for that matter, you need to know how fast it beats while you lift weights.) If you know that your exercise has not elevated your heart rate into your target zone, you can increase the effort you're putting into your cardiovascular activity to raise your heartbeat.

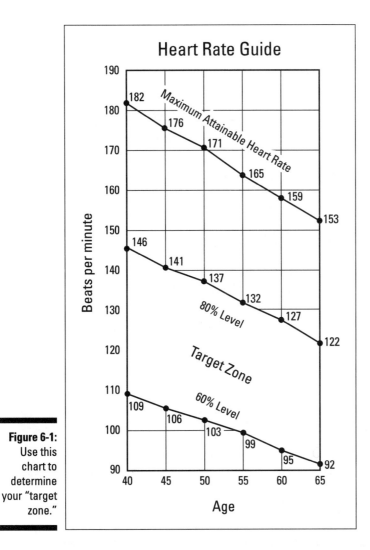

Figure 6-1:
Use this chart to determine your "target zone."

Most exercise machines (even those built for the home-equipment market) have a heart rate monitor in the electronic display. You grasp a metallic sensor, and the heart rate monitor immediately palpates your pulse. This allows you to monitor how fast your heart is beating without stopping on your treadmill, stair stepper, or stationary bike.

If you rely on walking through the neighborhood or thrice-weekly tennis games to raise your heart level, you should still monitor your heart rate to make sure that you're reaching the target zone. You can accomplish this in a low-tech way or a high-tech way.

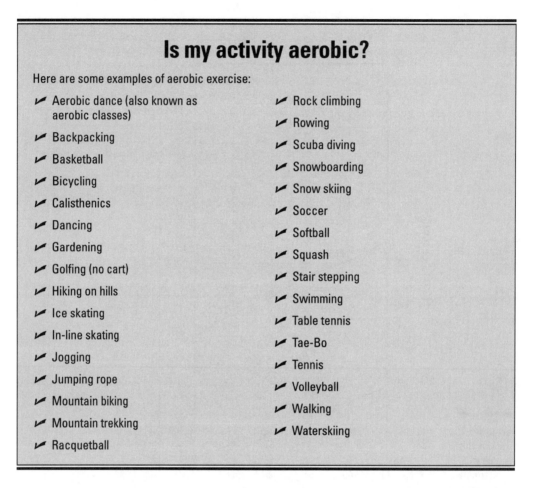

Is my activity aerobic?

Here are some examples of aerobic exercise:

- Aerobic dance (also known as aerobic classes)
- Backpacking
- Basketball
- Bicycling
- Calisthenics
- Dancing
- Gardening
- Golfing (no cart)
- Hiking on hills
- Ice skating
- In-line skating
- Jogging
- Jumping rope
- Mountain biking
- Mountain trekking
- Racquetball
- Rock climbing
- Rowing
- Scuba diving
- Snowboarding
- Snow skiing
- Soccer
- Softball
- Squash
- Stair stepping
- Swimming
- Table tennis
- Tae-Bo
- Tennis
- Volleyball
- Walking
- Waterskiing

- The **low-tech** way is pausing during exercise and placing three middle fingers over the radial artery of the wrist. For those of you who stayed as far away as you could from high school anatomy class (like me), you locate the radial artery by turning your palm upward and placing three fingers on the wrist just before it joins with the hand. Count the beats for ten seconds, and then multiply by six to compute the current pulse.

The problem with taking your pulse manually is the awkward coordination involved in looking at your watch and counting beats when your wrist is turned over with three fingers resting on the radial artery. Trust me: Seeing your timepiece and counting the beats accurately in a ten-second time frame is not easy. Another point is that after you stop exercising to take your pulse, your heartbeat starts to drop rapidly. If you have to recount two or three times, you've lost the benefit.

✔ The **high-tech** way is purchasing a wristwatch heart rate monitor that comes with a wireless transmitter inside a comfortable elastic band that you strap around your chest. Perhaps you've seen a shirtless man running on the side of the road with a strap around his chest; he was wearing a heart rate monitor. The strap picks up the direct electrical impulses of the heart and transmits the results to the wrist receiver. The readings are highly accurate — the same accuracy as an electro-cardiograph. The wrist receiver also acts like a sports watch, loaded with features: time of day, calendar, alarm, calorie counter, and a PC interface that can transfer recorded training data to your personal computer for analysis.

Like anything in this computerized world, these heart monitor gizmos have come *way* down in price. You can find excellent models for under $100. Several top brands are Polar (`www.polarusa.com`), Acumen (`www.acumeninc.com`), and Cardiosport (`www.cardiosport.com`).

One drawback about these heart monitors is that you have to wear a strap around your chest while you exercise. I think a better alternative is handheld pulsemeters, which you hold in your hand, stick in your pocket, or affix to a piece of equipment. The heart rate monitor reads your pulse from your fingertip and displays the results digitally. Hand-held pulsemeters are cheaper; many can be found for under $50.

Don't forget that your goal in all of this is to get inside your target heart range and stay there for at least 20 minutes. Do this three times a week, and you are well on the road to having a healthy heart.

The Fitness Heavyweight: Anaerobic Exercise

Now turn your attention to anaerobic exercise, which is usually accomplished through using strength-training machines such as Nautilus or Hoist or by lifting free weights — dumbbells and barbells raised without the guidance of a machine. (See Chapter 7 for more on exercise equipment.) But you don't have to lift weights to get some anaerobic exercise. Body weight exercises such as sit-ups, push-ups, or pull-ups can suffice.

However you do it, just do it (sorry, Nike!). To lose weight and become fit when you're over 40, *you must add anaerobic exercise to your fitness regimen.*

The seven fittest sports

Mirror, mirror, on the wall,

Who's the fittest of them all?

The Fairy Godmother would answer, "Cross-country skiers, of course!"

In real life, considerable debate rages among exercise physiologists regarding which sport produces the fittest athletes. Physiologists generally measure fitness by five parameters: cardiovascular efficiency, body composition, strength/power, agility, and flexibility. Some sports require more of one than the other, which is why identifying the sport that brings human beings to their highest levels of fitness is largely an arbitrary and subjective exercise.

These seven sports, in no particular order after the first one, are head and shoulders above others in terms of fitness:

Cross-country skiing

Cross-country skiers rule the cardio roost. Physiologists have measured the aerobic capacity of world-class athletes to measure the maximal oxygen consumption (or VO_2 max), and cross-country skiers suck wind like no one else. As a way of comparison, a superbly conditioned soccer player would produce a VO_2 max of about 60 milliliters (ml) per kilogram of body weight per minute. I know this is all technical stuff, but it's rare for elite athletes to crack the 70 ml mark. When you put Norwegian or Swedish Olympic cross-country skiers to the test, they record values in the low 90s. Researchers believe this happens because the arms are a vital component of the cross-country stroke, as opposed to just using the legs when running.

Rowing

Rowers use their arms even more than cross-country skiers, but not their legs, which explains why they can't quite match the athletic prowess

of cross-country skiers. Yet in almost every other area — cardio, body composition, power, and agility — rowers take second seat to almost no one.

Cycling

Lance Armstrong, whom I admire so much for coming back from testicular cancer to win the Tour de France in 1999 and 2000, is said to have a resting heart rate of 33 beats a minute. That's even lower than tennis's Bjorn Borg was alleged to have, which was in the 40s. To give you an example of how fit Lance is, he can produce an incredible amount of power in his legs — and sustain it. Lance can pump those pedals to produce 500 watts of power throughout a 30-minute hill climb. I could sustain 500 watts of power for only about 30 seconds.

Canoeing and kayaking

Canoers and kayakers produce aerobic and power readings similar to runners and cyclists, but they don't even use their legs. It just goes to show you how much strength is needed to pull an oar through water.

Gymnastics

Don't let those 85-pound bodies fool you. Gymnasts don't have any weak muscles in their bodies. Everything gets used, which accounts for why they have ridiculously low body fat measurements of 2–4 percent. About the only area in which gymnasts do not score well is aerobic tests. Gymnasts are built of rock-hard muscle, although they do little or no weight training. They develop their muscles by lifting their own body weight during marathon training sessions.

Wrestling

I'm talking about real wrestling, not those awful Stone Cold Steve Austin rumbles seen Monday nights on TNT. Wrestlers are in fantastic shape because they wed aerobic and anaerobic exercise during their three-minute tussles. They run long distances, bench press hundreds of pounds, perform sit-ups and push-ups by the hundreds, and stretch for hours. It's enough to make you want to puke.

Water polo

Because most people watch water polo once every four years when the Olympic Games are on, they have no appreciation for how tough this sport is. Water polo appears to be all about pushing and shoving, but underneath the water's surface, those legs are churning like pistons.

The advantages of anaerobic exercise

Many studies have shown that anaerobic exercise burns more calories and thus more fat than aerobic exercise — up to *five* times more, according to a Colorado State University study. The results of that study are presented in Table 6-1.

Table 6-1	Calories Burned in 60 Minutes of Exercise		
Exercise	*During Exercise*	*2 Hours after Exercise*	*3–15 Hours after Exercise*
Aerobic	210	25	0
Anaerobic	650	150	260

Source: Dr. Christopher Melby of the Department of Food, Science, and Human Nutrition, Colorado State University, 1993.

As you can see, these types of exercises result in a huge difference in caloric expenditures. What happens is that aerobic exercise typically burns 25 percent muscle and 75 percent fat for body energy, but anaerobic exercise burns 100 percent body fat for body energy.

In addition, anaerobic exercise strengthens and develops muscle tissue, and this can increase your metabolism. Your body expends a lot of energy just to maintain and repair muscle tissue; even while you are asleep, your body is burning calories to take care of its muscles. In other words, the more muscle you have, the more calories your body needs just to exist.

Pay attention to this next point: People who do *not* engage in anaerobic exercise as they get older will lose muscle and bone mass, slow their metabolism, gain fat (stored surplus calories), and experience the deterioration of their internal organs and cardiovascular system.

You're not going to bulk up

When I first started working out in the weight room, I worried that I was going to "bulk up" too much — become muscle bound. Not only did I not want that look, but I believed that big muscles would interfere with the precise stroke production that I needed on the tennis court.

Since then, I've learned that women will not get bulging muscles because the male hormones just aren't present to jump-start that process. Those female bodybuilders you see on ESPN with those glistening muscles and Mr. Atlas poses got that way by taking hormone supplements and going crazy in the gym with super-intensive workouts.

As for those who believe that women's bodies are too frail to perform resistance exercise, I ask: What physical activity is more demanding than childbirth? Strength training is a safe and effective exercise for women. Your muscles won't balloon like some cartoon character, but you will develop strong and shapely muscles that are fit and functional.

Keep this in mind, too: Unless you do incorporate some type of resistance strength training into your exercise schedule, you will lose a half pound of muscle for every year past the age of 20. Even if you *still* weigh the same as you did 20 years ago, you've probably replaced 10 to 12 pounds of muscle with 10 to 12 pounds of fat. While aerobic exercise helps burn excess fat, strength training is the only remedy to build muscle.

Regarding bone mass, strength training cannot turn back the clock on osteoporosis after you have it, but recent research shows that regular strength training does maintain bone mass. It can even help those suffering from certain types of arthritis and chronic back pain.

Anaerobic exercise in the form of lifting weights gives us the muscular strength to go through life with a minimum of discomfort and lower risk of injuries. Expending the effort *today* to build and maintain strength should give you the ability to live independently and function normally for years to come.

Once may be enough

Weight training shouldn't be too much work. Pushing plates at your local health club twice a week for 30 minutes at a time is a good start. Three times a week would be superior for those making a lifestyle change. I can tell you this: You don't have to lift weights four or more times a week unless you're planning a World Wrestling Federation tryout.

I've always wondered this about strength work: How many reps? How frequently should I push those plates, lift that set of weights, curl that dumbbell? Is more better than less? If a set of ten is good for you, is a set of 20 better?

Not necessarily, according to a University of Florida study reported in *Medicine and Science in Sports and Exercise* in January 2000. An average person using free weights (such as barbells) or weight machines does not appear to derive any extra benefit by repeating a set of lifts several times.

Here's the kicker: **One set of repetitions should be enough.** (But be sure to use a weight that is challenging for the last two or three repetitions.)

Doing one set of reps is a great way to squeeze in a workout when you're pressed for time. A lunchtime workout — 20 minutes in the gym, 20 minutes on the bike, and ten minutes in the shower — is ample time for a one-hour lunch break. For those trying to work out between the end of work and dinner, a 20-minute run-through with the weights is sure better than nothing.

As for myself, I generally like to do a warm-up set at half my weight so I don't injure any muscles. I may do another set at 75 percent of my intended weight, and then I do my intended set. This works for me; experiment with what works best for you.

A little advice on weight training

Strength training does not have to be excessively strenuous. You see improvements in your fitness and strength right away. Follow these tips as you prepare for a strength-training regimen:

- **Leave the power lifting for the young bucks.** Check your egos at the door. They are younger and stronger than you. You have experience on your side.

- **Listen to your body.** If something doesn't feel right, stop what you're doing. Don't finish your set of repetitions. The "no pain, no gain" statement is false and can be dangerous.

- **You will not be able to do spot reduction.** Some people believe that if they work their flabby midsections, the pounds will melt away where they need it most. Sorry, but when you exercise, you use energy produced by burning fat in all parts of your body, not from the muscles doing the work. But you do lose weight across the board.

- **Your muscles will not turn to fat if you stop lifting weights.** Exercise cessation doesn't mean that the muscle tissue will turn into fat, because fat and muscle are totally different types of tissue. If you stop exercising (and I hope you won't), you have to cut back on the calories you consume. That's hard! I vote to continue exercising.

Aerobic versus anaerobic: An example

If you're having trouble understanding the difference between aerobic and anaerobic exercise, perhaps a word picture will help.

Suppose that you've been exercising on a stationary bike all winter long at your fitness club. Your usual routine is to pedal two or three times a week for 30-minute stints. Spring is in the air, so you decide to take advantage of the warm sun by going on an outdoor bike ride. The temperature is just right on this Saturday morning — around 70 degrees. It feels good to pedal briskly in the fresh air on a level bike path. You are performing classic aerobic exercise.

In the distance, you spot a series of hills. You pedal over the first one with little exertion, but you can feel it in your legs on the second hill. The final climb, however, is a killer: To keep up your cadence and speed, you stand on your pedals and give that little extra oomph to clear the rise.

What you've just done on Hill #3 is switch over from aerobic to anaerobic exercise. You handled the first two hills aerobically, but to maintain speed on the final rise, you needed extra help. When you stood on the pedals and pumped those tired leg muscles, you crossed a threshold and began exercising the body *anaerobically.* Chances are you couldn't sustain that type of energy exertion for very long, because only elite athletes can do *any* form of anaerobic exercise beyond a few moments. Yet anaerobic exercise is very good for you, and you need to find ways to include some in your weekly exercise schedule.

The Forgotten Exercise: Stretching

I can assure you that you'll never go wrong by stretching before working out or playing a sport. You should even stretch before you start your day job because the improved circulation and greater range of motion will allow you to go about your daily tasks feeling better.

That's why stretching needs to be seen as part of a three-legged fitness stool that includes cardiovascular endurance (aerobics) and strength (anaerobics) as the other two legs. Unfortunately, stretching is easy to overlook because most individuals (present company included) perceive stretching to be tedious, boring exercise that's uncomfortable and downright painful.

A few years ago, I met a man named Fred Dolan at a golf tournament in Florida. After a few minutes of small talk, I learned that Fred is the executive director of the American Flexibility Institute. I also learned that if I ever needed an evangelist for stretching, Fred is it.

"Stretching is all about improving the body's flexibility, but you need to understand why a stretching program is such a good thing for you," Fred says. "Stretching decreases the risk of injury, improves performance, and reduces muscle soreness following exercise."

Hey, golfers!

Listen up, golfers. I know who you are — the guys in the loud pants and colorful shirts. You probably think all this stretching stuff is for sissies, but a comprehensive stretching program can improve your clubhead speed by 6 percent! Do you know what that means? You could get 20 more yards off your drive and take a club less on your approach shots. Pros would give their first child to increase their clubhead speed by that amount. Stretching sounds like a good deal to this neophyte golfer!

According to Fred, these are the primary goals of stretching:

✔ To achieve the proper balance of flexibility between opposing muscle groups

✔ To increase the range of motion of a body part without decreasing its strength or stability

✔ To increase the length of the muscle fibers without overstretching the associated tendons and ligaments

That may not mean much to some of you, so I'll boil it down: Stretching is good. Allow me to amend this: Stretching is *very* good for you. Stretching increases circulation and blood flow, relaxes the body, and improves coordination. You feel mentally alert, and your anxiety and stress are reduced. After you become more flexible, your body is less prone to injury, enjoys a greater range of motion, recovers from workouts more quickly, and just feels better.

I agree that stretching is not exciting or filled with thrills, but you still need to stretch anyway. Look at stretching the way you look at flossing your teeth: It's not a pleasant chore, but you're going to prevent a whole host of problems down the road. Some exercise books and fitness gurus counsel stretching for 15–30 minutes, but this is not realistic. Many of us cannot make the time commitment to stretch that long. But we can certainly stretch for several minutes before exercising or playing a sport.

Guys should know this about stretching: You need it more than women do. Men generally have less flexibility than women do because women have more of the muscle protein elastin, which promotes muscle flexibility.

Chapter 7

The Skinny on Exercise Machines

*T*oday's exercise machines are high-tech horses that you can jump on and ride comfortably while you pursue a workout *par excellence.* The hottest exercise machines these days are called "ellipticals" because they simulate walking, stepping, and cycling with an elliptical, low-impact motion while your arms work synchronized levers for a total body workout. (I'll have more to say about elliptical machines later.)

Any exercise machine is apt to be cutting edge these days, however, because the burgeoning fitness market has given companies incentive to innovate and improve their lines of treadmills, exercise bikes, stair steppers, and so on. The latest development — and one you're going to be seeing more of in coming years — is exercise machines equipped with built-in computer screens that allow you to tap into the Internet, read your e-mail, or even watch *I Love Lucy* reruns. Meanwhile, even the humblest exercise machine comes with a reading rack so you can pass the time with a magazine or a novel that you never had time to finish.

This chapter gives an overview of the various machines found in many health clubs today and offers a few pros and cons regarding each machine. After reading this chapter, you'll have a better understanding of what kind of exercise machine (or machines) will be best for you.

Determining Your Apparatus Status

I'm assuming that you want to use an exercise machine to raise your heart rate, break into a sweat, and work your upper and lower body. No matter which machine you decide to adopt as your "main event," however, just about any machine helps you burn calories by the bushel, shapes and tones your body, or delivers a heart-boosting cardiovascular workout if you stay on it long enough.

When choosing the right machine, you should be looking for one that suits your interests and is enjoyable and easy to use. After all, if exercising isn't fun, you don't have much incentive to return to the gym the next day or 48 hours later. Someone's favorite machine, however, could be your instrument of torture. For example, your aching knees may protest a stair stepper but heartily approve of a recumbent stationary cycle, in which the rider is in a reclining position with the legs extended in front of the body. Your back may hurt after 15 minutes of rowing, but you may welcome the rhythmic walking found on a treadmill. Only you can decide which machine "feels" right.

What are your long-range goals? If you're trying to lose weight, for example, then you'll want to evaluate the calorie expenditures. Machines that combine upper- and lower-body exercise (such as dual-action bikes, rowing machines, and elliptical machines) burn more calories per minute and increase your heart rate sooner. Exercising more muscle groups at one time means a higher-intensity workout. Don't forget that 30 percent of your muscles are located in your upper body, but those muscles receive little exertion while you're striding on a treadmill or churning your legs on an exercise bike.

You also need to find out which muscles the machine emphasizes. Your muscles may tire before you reach your target heart rate, or you may find that a stair-climbing machine builds up your calves (located in the back of the lower legs) when you really wanted to exercise your gluteals (your rear end).

Get That Blood Pumping: Aerobic Exercisers

People love options, and you certainly have them when it comes to choosing aerobic exercise equipment that's right for you. (See Chapter 6 for a description of aerobic and anaerobic exercise.) If you haven't ridden a stationary bike in years, your buns will notice the anatomically designed seats in the newer models. Some of the new "self-generating" exercise bikes come loaded with a computer chip that automatically adjusts the machine's resistance to keep your heart in the fat-burning zone, which is 60 to 80 percent of your maximum heart rate. (See Chapter 6 for more on heart rates). As you walk your fingers through this list, don't be afraid to try something new.

Treadmills

Treadmills are getting lots of mileage these days, and for good reason. Treadmills go at your pace, although most people use them to pace their walking, not jogging. People like treadmills for their predictability — the reliable roll of the belt, the comfortable indoor temperature, and the *Seinfeld* reruns airing on the overhead TV. Many have display monitors that can hold magazines or newspapers and a cradle for a water bottle.

All treadmills provide a manual mode that allows participants to mix a variety of speeds and inclines at will. You step on the deck, punch in some commands and numbers on the display monitor, and off you go. Some offer the "Broderick Crawford," an exercise named after the gravelly voiced star of the old *Highway Patrol* TV series. The "Broderick Crawford" has a "10-4" pattern: warm up for ten minutes, increase speed for ten minutes, slow down for ten minutes, and then finish strong for ten minutes.

Treadmills come with handrails, but those should be renamed "safety bars" because most people rarely touch the rails during their half hour or hour of walking. Many treadmill users naturally swing their arms while striding so they can earn an upper-body workout as well. (See Figure 7-1.)

Pros: The treadmill, which allows you to walk indoors in a climate-controlled, safe environment, delivers more exercise than you'd think. According to the *Journal of the American Medical Association,* treadmills easily outpace exercise bikes and rowing machines when it comes to calories burned per hour.

Cons: You need discipline — or something good to watch on TV — to stay motivated. Because treadmills are the most popular exercise equipment in fitness clubs, you may be hard-pressed to find a free one during the after-work rush.

Stationary bikes

Stationary bikes may not travel anywhere, but like their outdoor cousins, they are extremely efficient in generating health benefits. A 22-minute, moderate intensity workout on a stationary exercise bike will burn 150 calories in a 150-pound person. Burning an extra 150 calories most days of the week is the prescription for sedentary individuals to achieve significant health improvements, according to the "Surgeon General's Report on Physical Activity and Health."

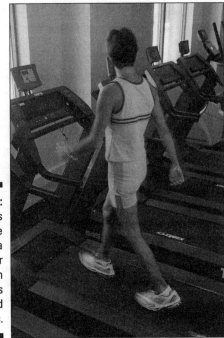

Figure 7-1:
Treadmills
have
become a
popular
fixture in
fitness
centers and
homes.

Another big advantage of riding indoors, besides shielding yourself from the raw elements, is the ability to monitor your pulse rate. You also don't have to worry about getting nailed by an automobile or someone opening a car door as you're about to pass by. Those of us over 40 feel comfortable riding a stationary bike because most of us rode bikes as kids. Exercise bikes have the lowest learning curve of any piece of fitness equipment on a gym room floor.

They also are easy on the body — especially the new *recumbent* versions, which retain the pedal action but substitute a chair-like seat and back for the old familiar saddle on upright bikes. (See Figure 7-2.) Recumbent bikes are ideal for those with back pain or those who are severely overweight. The recumbent position distributes weight more evenly over the lower back and buttocks because the seat supports the entire pelvis and lumbar spine. They are ideal for cardiac rehabilitation because the heart does not have to fight as much gravity to pump blood. Handicapped individuals and seniors with balance problems will find recumbents easier to use.

Two other, more traditional styles of bikes are available:

- ✔ Upright bikes most resemble the action felt when you bicycle.
- ✔ Dual-action bikes are upright stationary bikes that use air resistance or attachments to work your arms.

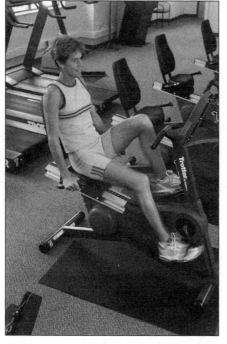

Figure 7-2:
Betsy
using a
recumbent
exercise
bike, which
is easier
on the
back than
traditional
upright
bikes.

The dual-action models are the only ones that give you an upper-body work-out. With upright and recumbent bikes, your arms are essentially taking a siesta.

Stationary bikes use brake-pad, strap-resistance, and air-resistance technolo-gies these days. Brake-pad bikes, which have a weighted flywheel and a system of brake calipers regulated by resistance, are lowest in cost. Strap-resistance bikes employ a nylon strap that tightens and loosens around a weighted flywheel. Air-resistance bikes, such as the Schwinn Airdyne, use spinning fan blades to create resistance; the faster you pedal, the higher the resistance and the greater the work (no fair!). But the fanning action of the flywheel blades cools you.

My recommendation is that you try a dual-action bike, which packs a calorie-eating wallop. But if you're the adventurous type, or used a road bike in your youthful days, you just have to try a new kind of exercise bike making its way into clubs these days — a *spinner* bike.

Spinners are sleek, road-race versions of the stationary bike. Spinner bikes have some extra features: a pedal-resistance control knob that riders use to make quick adjustments; toe clips so riders can receive maximum pedaling efficiency; multiposition handlebars, which provide for a variety of hand and arm positions; and a water bottle cage for hydration. What you *won't* find is an on-board computer.

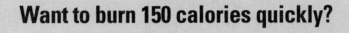

Want to burn 150 calories quickly?

Here's how long you would have to work out in a gym to burn 150 calories (if you weigh around 150 pounds):

✔ 17 minutes while jogging slowly on a treadmill at 5 mph

✔ 21 minutes while using a stair stepper at a moderate pace

✔ 21 minutes while doing the circuit on strength-training machines

✔ 22 minutes while riding a stationary bike with moderate resistance at 10 mph

✔ 27 minutes while walking on a treadmill at 4 mph

Pros: Exercise bikes come in so many variations that it's almost impossible not to find one you like. They've even come out with dual-action versions so you can receive a total-body workout.

Cons: Some people find it monotonously difficult to keep the legs churning.

Stair steppers

Stair steppers are cardiovascular machines that deliver an excellent aerobic workout and toning for the lower body. They aren't for people with bad knees, such as myself, or someone with a history of back problems. But stair steppers are a low-impact alternative to jogging or running. Many women worry that steppers will balloon their legs, hips, and buttocks. But that's not true. Stair steppers will tone those problem areas as you burn calories and lose fat. (See Figure 7-3.)

Exercisers need to pay attention to several things when using stair steppers. One of the biggest gym sins is using the arms to support the body's weight — leaning on the handrails while the legs struggle to keep up. This posture places extra stress on the lower back, shoulders, elbows, and wrists, and doesn't give the legs nearly the workout you bargained for.

"Leaners" must switch to the manual mode and lessen the intensity readings immediately. Correct your body position by standing up straight with your upper body in the same vertical plane as your hips and legs. The handrails should be lightly held for balance. Under this positioning, the large muscles in the legs will have to work to support all your weight, resulting in the expenditure of more calories and the construction of more muscle. Hyperextension injuries of the knee have been known to occur during the bottom of the pedal stroke, when the knee is fully extended, so warm up slowly. In fact, most injuries on stair steppers can be attributed to an inadequate warm-up period. Here's a good idea: Pedal five minutes on a stationary bike before mounting a stepper.

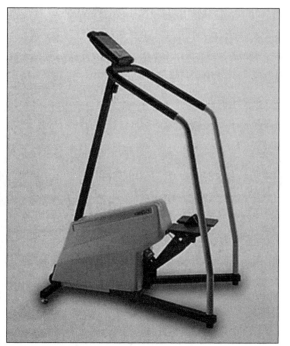

Figure 7-3:
Stair
steppers,
such as this
one by
Tectrix, are
a low-
impact
alternative
to jogging.

After an initial warm-up period, start the stair climber at a lower step rate and gradually work up to a stepping rate that will elevate your heart rate to a level within your target heart zone. Use the manual control button to alternate between a slower, deeper step routine and a quicker, shallower stepping motion.

I prefer *independent* steppers in which the pedals — also known as foot platforms — are not related to each other. When you push down on one leg, the other stays put until you take the weight off the first leg and push with the other leg. This action is more natural and provides a tougher workout. Some older (and less expensive) steppers have *dependent* action, which means the pedals are directly connected to one another. When you push down with one foot, the other comes up automatically. I think this gives way to herky-jerky movements.

Stair steppers come in two variations. The StairMaster Stepmill looks like a mini-escalator-in-a-machine. Then you have another climber that's similar to climbing a long 2x12-inch piece of wood 10 feet long. You have to be Rambo-tough to handle these climbers. You strap your feet in and then reach up to pull down — and push up on the handlebars that are placed at eye level or over your head while you step. The motion resembles climbing a ladder, and participants soon become exhausted.

Pros: You huff and puff while climbing story after story with these cardiovascular machines.

Cons: You can cheat on these machines by leaning on the handlebars. They are not ideal for those with knee and ankle problems.

Elliptical exercisers

A recent evolution in fitness machines has been the development of elliptical exercisers — a cross between an exercise bike and a ski machine, with a bit of stair climber thrown in for good measure. (See Figure 7-4.)Your feet loop forward while your hands grasp the handlebars (also known as pedal arms) that move in sync with your feet. This is known as a natural elliptical movement — standing on the machine, putting your feet in the foot pedals, grabbing the stick-like handlebars, and pumping like a piston. Not all elliptical machines come with pedal arms, so be sure to gravitate toward ellipticals that can offer a full-body workout with arm-motion levers that move fluidly while your legs pump elliptically.

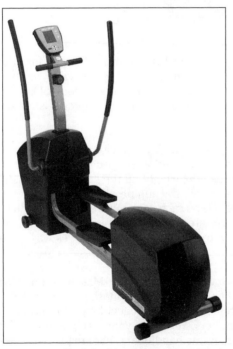

Figure 7-4:
Elliptical exercisers such as this Schwinn 400p Elliptical are a cross between an exercise bike and a ski machine.

Photo by Dennis Lane Photography, Denver, Colorado

The legs receive a strong workout from the up-and-down stepper motion as you stride. The arms receive a satisfactory upper-body workout as one arm shoots forward while the other pulls back. Many elliptical exercisers work in reverse, which means you can work different muscles and experience some variety while walking backward.

Ellipticals provide great low-impact exercise for people with knee problems, but those in superior physical condition usually find the machines too easy. I think elliptical trainers are best used for those change-of-pace days in the gym when you want to ride on something different.

Pros: Elliptical machines are the latest technological advance in fitness — a step above, so to speak, stair steppers. You receive a total body workout in no time at all with little or no impact on the body's joints. Health clubs say they rank second in popularity to treadmills.

Cons: They can be hard to find.

Cross-country ski trainers and rowing machines

I combined these two types of exercise machines because the demand for rowing machines and cross-country ski trainers — while never very large — is doing the incredible shrinking act.

Cross-country ski machines, popularized by NordicTrack before the company went bankrupt in 1998, require synchronized arm and leg movements and more coordination than treadmills, steppers, and exercise bikes. (The NordicTrack name has since been purchased by Icon Health & Fitness, which is using it to sell a line of ellipticals, exercise bikes, and ski machines.) Unless you grew up in a cold-weather climate and learned how to cross-country ski, you're going to find it difficult to glide your feet back and forth on roller-mounted boards or foot pads while your arms swing back and forth as your hands grip handles that are attached to ropes. Whew!

Rowing machines, while inherently simpler, are no day at the lakeshore either. You use your back, legs, and arms to row while you push the sliding seat backward and forward.

Pros: No one can deny that ski trainers and rowing machines offer strenuous cardiovascular workouts with push-pull motions that work many of the major muscle groups.

Cons: They are the most difficult exercise machines to use, and elliptical trainers in health clubs are replacing ski machines and rowers across the country.

Weighty Matters: Dumbbells, Barbells, and Strength Machines

Although aerobic fitness improves general health and endurance, most aerobic exercise does little to increase muscular strength. You need to add anaerobic exercise, which is why you should do some strength training on a weight machine or with free weights.

In case you're not sure about your fitness terms, *strength-training machines* (see Figure 7-5) are interesting-looking contraptions that you usually sit in or lie down on to work a group (or groups) of muscles against resistance so that the muscles become tired. The resistance can come in a number of forms: flat, weighted plates (usually in 10-pound increments); air cylinders; rubber tubing; or elastic bands. *Free weights* are dumbbells (see Figure 7-6) and barbells (see Figure 7-7) that are lifted without the external support of a machine. Dumbbells are small bars for single-arm exercises, while barbells are long bars used in two-arm exercises.

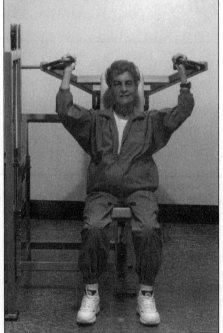

Figure 7-5: Weight-training machines, such as this shoulder press machine, build up muscle strength in different areas of the torso.

Free weights and weight machines build strength in three ways:

- ✔ **Resistance:** Resistance challenges the muscles to work harder than they are used to working, which causes them to contract with greater force and increase in size and strength. Added strength brings dramatic physical benefits, including the ability to perform many ordinary activities — such as climbing stairs or carrying groceries in from the car — with greater ease.

- ✔ **Repetition:** You have to repeat the resistance training an adequate number of times to benefit and to produce significant muscle fatigue. Tons of good news here: One set of repetitions or "reps" (eight to 12 times) is all you need on weight machines, although some people like to do two sets just to be sure.

- ✔ **Intensity:** You have to put something into it to get something back, but care must be given to not overdo it because you can easily injure yourself or become too sore. Body builders and other serious fitness folks say that you have to "feel the burn" when you lift, referring to the burning sensation that you feel when your muscles are screaming out under heavy exertion. Again, that's not true. The burn could be a signal that you're being *too* intense and that you need to back off a plate or two on the weight machine.

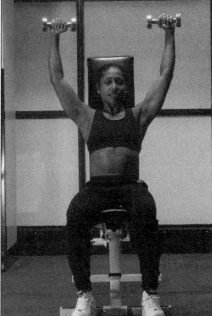

Figure 7-6:
Lifting a few dumbbells is a good way to round out your strength-training program.

Figure 7-7:
Barbells are used by people who have moved past the beginning stage of their weight-training program.

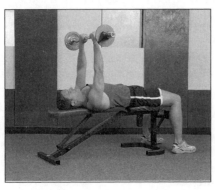

Welcome to the (strength) machine

You could purchase an expensive home gym as described in Chapter 10. But I think you're going to be better off joining a fitness center where you have a variety of strength machines at your disposal and trainers who can show you how to properly use those machines — and get the most out of them.

If you haven't darkened the door of a fitness gym in ten or 20 years, you're going to be surprised — and perhaps intimidated — by what you see on the main fitness floor. The padded strength-training machines resemble high-tech torture racks, and unless someone shows you how to get into one, you would be hard pressed to figure out what you're supposed to do after you're seated. But don't worry. Fitness trainers *love* to show members how the strength-training equipment works. Besides, club management won't allow you to start using the machines without a walk-through anyway — for liability reasons.

Strength-training machines are designed to target different sections of the torso, such as the

- Neck.
- Shoulders.
- Deltoids (the cap of the shoulders).
- Trapezius (upper portion of the back).
- Rhomboids (muscles in the middle of the upper back between the shoulder blades).
- Pectoralis major (large fan-shaped muscle that covers the front of the upper chest.
- Biceps (the front of the upper arm).
- Triceps (the back of the upper arm).

- ✔ Abdominals (stomach area).

- ✔ Lower back.

- ✔ Gluteals (the big muscle covering your butt).

- ✔ Quadriceps (the muscles in the front of the thigh).

- ✔ Hamstrings (the muscles in the back of the thigh).

- ✔ Hip abductors and adductors (the muscles of the inner and outer thigh).

- ✔ Calf (lower leg).

Different manufacturers produce strength-training machines. The brand name with the highest name recognition is Nautilus; you can't go wrong joining a club stocked with Nautilus machines. Cybex, Hoist, and Pace are other well-known strength-training machine companies.

After a trainer has shown you how to use the various machines, lift at a pace that works for you. You should not skip machines, because you want to receive a total body workout. Most people do the machines in roughly the same order, although you can certainly bounce around to different machines if one is taken when you're ready to get on.

If the last time you lifted weights was when President Reagan was in office, you should resume strength training with a light touch. Ladies, this means that you could go through the various Nautilus machines without using any weights at all on your first day back. See how that feels. If you try to lift too many plates the first time, you could have a tough time raising your arms the next morning to run a brush through your hair. You can add a plate or two a couple of days later. Remember that you can always add more weights later, but you can't reverse a torn muscle or some other injury.

Free the weights!

Often overlooked by getting-back-into-shape folks are the lowly free weights — those metal bars that have weighted plates welded or attached onto the ends. You're probably more familiar with dumbbells, the short, shiny, chrome-plated free weights that you see lined up in pairs in a rack alongside the wall.

Lifting free weights will probably not be the centerpiece of your anaerobic exercise program, but you should try to round out your weight-training workout by at least lifting a few dumbbells. You can leave the larger barbells to the serious lifters who strut around the club with wide leather belts strapped around their midsections.

Start with pairs of dumbbells weighing 2.5, 5, or perhaps 10 pounds, although the latter weight is usually too much for beginners. Let your arms hang by your side with a dumbbell in each hand. Then lift both hands toward your shoulders, keeping your elbows tucked in and bent. Repeat this until your upper arms are tired.

Another good exercise is to hold your hands at your side and shrug your shoulders. Then you can lift one arm straight out from your body. A personal trainer can show you a dozen more strength-training exercises that can be accomplished with dumbbells. Just be sure to put the dumbbells back in the rack when you're done!

Chapter 8

Exploring the Gym Jungle

. . . .

. . . .

*A*fter you've determined your fitness level, stopped ordering extra sour cream on your *chalupas*, shopped for your first Supplex/Lycra outfit, and resolved to shed excess poundage, you wonder: *What do I do next?*

For many people, signing on the dotted line and joining a fitness gym is the best way to get fit and stay fit. Nearly 30 million Americans belong to some kind of health club. Other options are available, of course, which involve working out at your place of employment (corporate fitness centers) or working out in the comfort of your own home; I cover those fitness avenues in Chapters 9 and 10. But this chapter helps you decide whether joining a fitness facility will help you meet your goals, gives you tips on evaluating health clubs and other fitness centers, and presents you pointers on choosing the one that best meets your needs.

Change of Venue: Deciding Whether to Join a Fitness Center

Deciding whether to join a fitness club is a tough call for many people. First, you must answer this key question: *Will I have time to use the health club?* If your answer is yes and you've determined that a monthly health club bill won't bust your budget, you're ready to weigh the other considerations.

Most importantly, the exercise facility must meet your fitness needs. If your exercise program consists solely of walking, a club may not be best for you. You can walk in your neighborhood for free, or purchase a treadmill for the amount of money you would probably spend for a year or two of club membership.

But if you're also looking to push a few strength-training machines around after your treadmill workout, you'll probably want to join a bare-bones gym. However, if you like to play racquetball, take in an aerobics class, hire a personal trainer, or sip a protein power shake while watching a big-screen *Monday Night Football* game, then you'll want a full-service health club. Expect to pay more for these amenities, however.

Think through what type of club that you want to join. If you're not a swimmer, but the club has the fanciest indoor pool in the state, you could be paying extra in monthly dues to heat a pool that you're not going to use. And you'll find a world of difference between a tennis club with fitness facilities and a fitness center with tennis courts. I wouldn't want to join the latter because tennis is a sideline activity there; I couldn't count on finding any serious tennis players. If I joined a tennis club with a well-stocked gym, however, I would enjoy plenty of competition on the courts, and I could do my workout after my tennis game.

Fitness to Be Tried: Your Health Club Choices

If you're considering joining a fitness club, you may be surprised at the number of choices in this area. The International Health, Racquet & Sportsclub Association (IHRSA) reports more than 12,000 commercial health clubs nationwide, but they vary in size and scope. Take a closer look at your alternatives:

- **All-purpose, everything-under-one-roof fitness emporiums or "sports clubs,"** such as Bally Total Fitness and L.A. Fitness, have strength-training machines by the score, tightly packed rows of treadmills and steppers, gleaming racquetball and basketball courts, steam rooms, spas, saunas, whirlpools, lap pools, aerobics classes, cardio kickboxing classes, dance lessons, personal trainers, masseuses, tanning machines, yoga classes, tai-chi classes, child care facilities, juice bars, bakeries, and restaurants. The list could go on: Some high-end clubs offer water slides, tennis and squash courts, hitting nets for golfers, baseball batting cages, rock climbing walls, and indoor running tracks, all amid modernistic stainless steel fixtures and curved stairways.

- **Community centers,** either municipally run or operated by private organizations (for example, Jewish Community Centers), have considerably fewer amenities, but you can usually find a decent gym and a multipurpose room used for Jazzercise classes or basketball games.

- **YMCAs** have something for everyone, including family rates. The machines may not be state-of-the-art and the facilities may be spartan, but you'll discover the setup to be more than adequate. More than 2,000 YMCAs and YWCAs can be found around the country.

- ✔ **Tennis and golf clubs** have added workout facilities in recent years. Even venerable country clubs more known as "social clubs" are recognizing the value that a fitness room brings to its members.

- ✔ **Storefront gyms,** found in mini-malls or in business districts, are considerably smaller than the "big box" fitness centers. They offer low prices, basic facilities, and personalized service.

- ✔ More **hotel fitness clubs** are opening their facilities to the public. You can count on a swimming pool and several machines tucked away in a room, but not much more.

- ✔ Hospitals and HMOs operate **wellness centers** that are part rehab, part fitness facilities. Nearly all wellness centers are open to the public for a monthly fee (in other words, you don't have to be a patient of the hospital or a member of the HMO). You won't find "Spandex bunnies" hopping from machine to machine, however. You're more likely to see older people trying to work themselves back into shape.

- ✔ Some big-name personal trainers own and operate fully equipped **private gyms** that clients use by appointment under the trainers' watchful eyes.

- ✔ Last, but not least, **specialty gyms** cater to niche markets, such as body builders and women only.

Wellness centers may be a good fit

You wouldn't necessarily associate hospitals and fitness centers in the same sentence, but more and more health care facilities are opening "wellness centers" that put plenty of medical muscle behind their mission statement. These fitness centers, located on-site at more than 550 hospitals and medical clinics around the country, are complete exercise facilities with all the treadmills, steppers, and strength-training machines found elsewhere.

Several things set wellness centers apart. The clientele is apt to be older and more genteel. In other words, you won't see WWF wrestlers lifting weights here on their days off. The staff is comprised of qualified medical professionals. You also won't see high school kids administering fitness assessment tests; at most wellness centers, certified exercise physiologists give heart, lung, and stress tests to new members, and then prepare a workout regimen. Physical therapy services are available, and cardiologists are on-call with defibrillators, just in case anyone slumps over on the exercise bike. The line between medical rehabilitation and fitness often blurs at wellness centers, but if you're fine with that distinction, you shouldn't have a problem. The larger centers put together programs for patients who have already had in-hospital cardiac or pulmonary rehabilitation or physical therapy for osteoporosis or musculo-skeletal injuries and surgery.

Wellness centers charge extra for these services, putting their initiation fees and monthly dues in line with high-end clubs. Many wellness centers are open to the public for a monthly fee, although in some larger cities, you must have a doctor's referral before you can join (which means your health insurance may cover the club fees).

Remember, though, that some or many of these options may not be available where you live. The Yellow Pages (look under "Health Clubs") are the first place to look for a club in your area; an Internet search could elicit much of the same information. Ask friends and neighbors for the name of a good club.

Finding the right fitness venue is all about trial and error, determining what you want out of a club, and looking for a place that fits your lifestyle, budget, and exercise preferences. Never join a club without taking them up on a trial membership (usually several days or one week at no charge).

The Club Tour Checklist

After you decide that your fitness program can really benefit from joining a health club or similar facility, visit ones in your area (see "Location, Location, Location" later in this chapter). When you tour a fitness club that you're thinking of joining, evaluate it in each of the following categories:

✔ **What's the overall facility like?**

- **Age and equipment selection:** Is this a well-rounded gym with the latest machines? Or does everything look a bit worn? Are the locker rooms adequate? Can you lock your valuables and store your clothes in a locker?

- **Cleanliness:** Are the machines "icky" and not wiped down periodically? Does the carpet look like it had better days — in 1979? What are the shower and locker room facilities like? Do they resemble a frat house on Sunday morning?

- **Parking:** Do you have to park on the street and walk in the dark, or is free, convenient parking available close to the front door?

- **Swimming pool:** Is the water warm enough? Does the pool have enough lanes to handle the swimming traffic? Do they close the entire pool during water aerobics classes, or are some lanes left open for swimmers? Is the pool deep enough?

- **Ambience:** Do you feel comfortable with the mix of people? Does the club cater to the twenty-something singles crowd, or are all ages represented? Do you see plenty of gray hairs?

✔ **What's inside?**

- **Equipment:** What strength-training machines are on the floor? Are you familiar with them? What time constraints are put on how long you can stay on a particular machine — a stationary bike, for example?

- **Crowdedness:** Is the club overrun during peak times — 5–7 p.m.? Will you have to wait to use a machine? Would it be worth it to pay more and join a more expensive club with fewer members?

- **Classes:** Are different aerobic classes available for you to take? Are the classes given at convenient times compatible with your work schedule? What about classes on nutrition, weight loss, and smoking cessation?

- **For women only:** Some clubs offer workout areas with treadmills, Nautilus machines, and free weights just for women. Is this important to you?

✔ **Who's there to help?**

- **Staffing:** Is adequate staffing available to answer questions and get help, or does one person staff the front desk, answer the phone, and sell products?

- **Fitness testing:** Will the club offer you a state-of-the-art physical assessment? Can you get a cholesterol screening?

- **Personal trainers:** If you want to take yourself to the next fitness level, are personal trainers available for consultation and planning? How skilled are they?

- **Feedback:** Does the club survey its membership to determine whether the members' interests and needs are being met?

✔ **How it will affect your bottom line?**

- **Dues:** What is the monthly membership fee? Do you have to come up with one lump sum for the whole year, or can you pay monthly or quarterly? Must you pay an initiation fee? (See "What You Can Expect to Pay" later in this chapter.)

- **Add-on fees:** Are you charged extra to use one of their towels? What about nutrition or aerobics classes? Does it cost more to play racquetball?

- **Guest fees:** If you want to bring a friend, what is the charge?

The rest of this chapter provides details on some of the more important and interesting features of health clubs and other fitness facilities.

Location, Location, Location

Like real estate, the most important aspect about joining a gym is location. If you don't live within a five- or ten-minute commute from your gym, you're not going to use that health club over the long run — no matter how good the facilities are. You're better off joining a small fitness facility in a mini-mall five minutes from home than signing up at a fancy health club across town, 20 minutes or 40 clogged blocks away. You may use that beautiful fitness center for a month or two or three, but statistics tell us that you're destined to become a fitness dropout.

The health club industry has a term for it: the "12 weeks/12 minutes" phenomenon. Their studies show that most people stick with an exercise resolution for 12 weeks before falling away if the fitness facility is further than a 12-minute drive. Other studies indicate that *half* of all people who join a gym stop going after six months, no matter how close or far they live from a club. This explains why sports clubs are constantly promoting and talking internally about "retention rates."

Because our focus is fitness for a lifetime, we can't stress enough that you must live near your health club — the closer the better — to continue exercising. Your health club must be on your way home from work or a short drive away from where you live — no more than a dozen minutes maximum. This is why location outweighs all other considerations.

Club Amenities

Once a health club has passed your white glove test, it's time to consider the amenities. Child care could be at the top of your list if you recently became a mother or father. If you need aerobics classes to motivate you, classes must be offered at convenient times. You may prefer one type of cardiovascular machine (such as a stair climber) over other brands. Before you tour a new club, make a mental list of what's important to you. Then pepper your host with questions about the following amenities listed in this section.

Machinery row

In my mind, the quality of the fitness equipment should make or break your club experience. You should see a wide variety of industrial strength cardiovascular equipment, such as

- ✔ Treadmills.
- ✔ Stationary bikes.
- ✔ Stair steppers.
- ✔ Elliptical machines.

Check out the strength-training machines and free weights. The three major brands are Nautilus, Hoist, and Cybex, all of which are excellent, although serious weight crunchers will tell you that they are different.

For more information on these and other machines, see Chapter 7.

Aerobics classes

Many people — particularly women — are interested in aerobics classes. Be sure to take part in several classes during your trial membership to determine whether the classes are given at a level that you can handle. Ask other members who the best instructors are, and ask club personnel whether the instructors are certified. Pay attention to the leader's energy level and expertise — and her age. Your comfort level may rise if the instructor is over 40. Finally, the aerobics studio should have a suspended hardwood floor, which is easier on the knees and joints. (Suspended floors are built on wooden supports, not concrete slabs, so they have more "give.")

Personal trainers

Every club has them — personal trainers who guide, show, exhort, motivate, educate, encourage, and stimulate you to physical levels that you never thought possible. I'm a great believer in PTs, or personal trainers, because I competed — and lost — against tennis players whose fitness level soared after personal trainers whipped them into shape.

The biggest drawback to trainers is cost: Most charge between $30 and $60 an hour, which means if you employ the services of a personal trainer twice weekly, eight times a month at $50 per workout, you'll receive a $400 add-on to your health club bill. That's more than a nice car payment.

If your budget can handle the extra expense, however, I highly recommend personal trainers, especially if you're treading the fitness comeback trail. Trainers can help you improve your fitness level quicker, reduce chances of injuring yourself, and motivate you in a million different ways.

Trainers aren't for slackers

Personal trainers break you out of your exercise norms and hold you accountable. You *have* to show up at the appointed time (unless you're willing to forfeit a $50 cancellation fee for standing up your PT). They won't let you slack off. They put you through a vigorous workout, track your progress, correct your form, come up with new and exciting ways to exercise, and help you accomplish your fitness goals. You get a better workout and end up making more progress than if you are on your own. Personal trainers help prevent injuries, because the most common training mistakes are related to technique. Many people have a tendency to use too much weight, resulting in poor form. Incorrect technique decreases strength gains and greatly increases the risk of injury.

A good personal trainer will work muscles that you never thought you had. But the soreness will feel good! Personal trainers are knowledgeable about different exercises, how to properly use the strength-training equipment, and how to work past your fitness plateaus and avoid boredom.

You are a candidate for personal trainers if you can answer yes to the following questions:

- ✔ Do you have trouble motivating yourself?

- ✔ Are you clueless about how to set up an exercise program or follow one?

- ✔ Do you desire maximum results in minimum time with a program specially designed for you?

- ✔ Do you have special medical needs, such as arthritis, diabetes, or obesity? (Personal trainers will design a safe, efficient program that will speed your recovery or help you reach your weight loss goals.)

- ✔ Have you been injured and are you trying to regain the fitness level you lost?

- ✔ Do you enjoy some company while working out? (Personal trainers say they are like hairdressers — they hear everything. Seriously, some people need a mentor, and personal trainers fit that bill.)

- ✔ Do you need someone to push you beyond your limits? (A certified personal trainer will not hurt you. He or she knows what your body is capable of taking.)

- ✔ Do you want to be nurtured or need some TLC? (Personal trainers will recognize your desire for nurturing.)

Finding the trainer who is right for you

The personal trainer field is not a male-denominated career path. Plenty of women have become PTs and done quite well. Please know, however, that all you need to call yourself a personal trainer is a business card. No regulatory or licensing agency governs the industry, and no law requires trainers to be certified, although many gyms require it. According to IDEA, an organization of health and fitness professionals, more than 65,000 people call themselves trainers in the U.S.

Remember that your trainer will be touching you and seeing you in all your sweaty glory, so you may want to consider a trainer who is the same sex as you. This is a hands-on profession, which means a good personal trainer will be placing his or her hands on certain portions of your anatomy and pushing you to "give me four more."

Finding a personal trainer should be easy: Ask friends for recommendations, and when you get a name, watch that person put someone else through the paces. You should interview your potential personal trainer, asking questions that can reveal why he (or she) got into the field, how he plans to improve your fitness, and what his credentials and educational background are. Consider the personal trainer's attitude, interpersonal skills, and appearance. Does he practice what he preaches?

Unless a trainer has specific training in subjects such as physical therapy or nutrition, he or she should be cautious in giving advice in these areas. Good trainers will recognize their limitations and how they relate to the well-being of their clients.

What You Can Expect to Pay

The dues structure can vary wildly from fitness venue to fitness venue. If you're joining a ritzy golf club with a gleaming gym, you could be paying tens of thousands of dollars for initiation and $300–500 a month in dues. On the other side of the scale, a storefront gym will ask for $22 a month and no initiation, or a hotel fitness site may charge you a modest daily rate each time you drop in.

Nearly all health clubs charge an initiation fee, although some clubs will waive the initiation when trying to boost membership rolls. The cost to join clubs is something like this:

- ✔ High-end clubs charge $500 and up for initiation, plus $75 for monthly dues.

- ✔ Mid-tier clubs charge $250 and up for initiation, plus $50 for monthly dues.

- ✔ No-frills clubs change around $100 for initiation, plus $25 to $35 for monthly dues.

Discounts are offered to couples and families.

Another consideration is the *type* of membership you purchase. Clubs have different levels. A base price may cover just use of the weight-training equipment, but you'd have to pay extra to take aerobics classes or play racquetball. Bally Total Fitness, for example, has *five* membership classes. It may take a while to sort out which one works for you. Ask questions so that you can make an informed decision.

Things can get sticky when signing contracts at sports clubs, which are staffed by commissioned sales people. These documents, filled with legalese, are naturally written in favor of the fitness facilities and promise to bring the wrath of God down on you if you don't pay. Ask what happens if you stop going — drop out. Ask for the cancellation fees to be spelled out for you — cancellation upon relocation, death, or disability. Verbal commitments must show up in writing.

Becoming a health club member is a little like buying a new car — you should have room for negotiating and haggling with the sales people, especially when the club is running a special (which happens every other day, it seems). You could be told that this is today's price and if you don't sign now, the offer will be taken off the table, which smacks of high-pressure tactics. Some clubs will not let you take home the contract to study.

Expect to be pushed to make a two- or three-year commitment, because health clubs know that more than half of enrollees quit going after six months. This is where you must exercise the greatest caution. In general, do not lock yourself into a long-term contract (longer than one year) unless you're absolutely sure that this is going to be your club for the foreseeable future, and you don't foresee moving. Ask what the finance charges are — the small print may state that you get hit with an 18 percent finance charge if you don't pay the first year's dues in full at time of signing. Some clubs may allow you to pay on a month-to-month basis, but that is always more costly than paying for a full year in advance. If you're not sure whether you want to make the commitment, ask if you can purchase a two-week trial membership.

Some national fitness chains, such as Bally, allow you to use their clubs in other cities. Check for details. Other health clubs offer reciprocal rights at out-of-town clubs. If you're a business traveler, this can be a real bonus.

You don't have to join a club to use one: Personal trainers with their own gyms charge you $50 and up per hour, but that includes use of the fitness equipment.

Hours and Atmosphere

As a general rule, the larger the club, the longer the club will be open each day. Don't assume, however, that fitness establishments such as 24 Hour Fitness are open 24/7 — some are not open around the clock. A mom-and-pop storefront exercise gym may close at 7 p.m. and be closed on weekends and holidays, which could preclude you from working out. It doesn't help your fitness when you belong to a club that you can't use because it's closed at the time you want to work out.

Another consideration is what time the group classes are held for aerobics, step aerobics, kickboxing, and so on. The classes must jive with your availability if you plan to participate.

Tapping into the E-Zone

A new health club wouldn't think of opening its doors today without a row of TVs suspended above the treadmills, stair steppers, and exercycles. Watching the CNN newsloop helps beat the tedium of pumping those legs for 30 minutes without visual stimulation. It was only a matter of time, however, before someone built a better entertainment mousetrap.

A couple of options are being implemented in health clubs today. One is called the E-Zone Personal Entertainment System, which features a bright, vivid screen positioned just in front of your treadmill, stepper, stationary bike, and so on. You wear a pair of wireless headphones and can watch whatever cable channel you desire, or listen to your favorite CDs and audiocassettes. The wireless headphones mean that you can also jump on Nautilus machines and still listen to motivating, upbeat music while you work out.

An emerging technology found on exercise machines incorporates a touch-screen display, an audio CD player, a full-screen TV feed, and a high-speed Internet connection. A company named Netpulse has developed broadband machines that can be attached to stationary bikes, steppers, and elliptical trainers. Each rider logs on to a personal account that allows highly targeted advertising to come to the screen (that's the catch), but you can surf the Web, read your e-mail, shop in the Netpulse mall, watch TV — or track your workout progress while you step and stride.

Netpulse is currently found in several hundred high-end gyms, but more than 2,000 health clubs are expected to have Netpulse by 2001.

When you walk into a club, you want to feel as though you belong — not the fitness equivalent of walking into an establishment and having everyone stop talking to stare at this total geek who just came through the front door. Some match-ups are no-brainers: If you're a guy, don't bother visiting a club called "Fitness Elite for Women." If you're soft and pudgy from years of physical inactivity, you won't feel comfortable at Gold's Gym, where Hulk Hogan look-alikes dressed in pumpkin-colored tank tops slam weights in intimidating fashion.

Pay attention to the dress code of the club you're thinking of joining. Some high-end clubs are sticklers in this — no cargo shorts, polo shirts, or regular pants. So if you're in the neighborhood and want to spin the pedals along Bike Row, you won't be allowed to work out unless you're wearing "work-out" clothes.

Staff personnel generate much of a club's atmosphere. It helps to be greeted by a friendly face at the front desk. Staff members should readily show you how to use the machines and answer questions. You should see plenty of people your age — and in the same shape as you.

For Ladies Only: Clubs Exclusively for Women

As more health clubs open, more are hanging out shingles that say, "For Women Only." IHRSA estimates that approximately 2,000 women-only fitness centers in the U.S. serve 2 million women.

I can certainly understand the rationale we women have when it comes to working out. Tight-fitting and revealing exercise clothes cause many women to feel self-conscious about their bodies. Psychologists have a name for it: "physique anxiety." The older and larger you are, the more you are apt to be comfortable only when working out among other women. Women may prefer single-sex fitness centers for these reasons:

✔ They are recovering from health or medical issues.

✔ They were victims of domestic violence and physical or sexual abuse.

✔ Their religion (Islam, for example) prohibits exercising in a coed setting.

Stepping into the breach are women-only clubs like Fitness Elite for Women, La Physique, Lady of America, and Naturally Women, which offer exercise classes by women and for women. Strength-training machines by Cybex and Pace are specially designed to fit a woman's body and come equipped with lighter weighted plates. Women can also find on-site dieticians, facials, body waxing, and massage therapy.

Women-only fitness clubs are ideal for "deconditioned" women who don't know a barbell from a dumbbell but have made the commitment to do something about their weight and physique while they still have time. If this description sounds like you, I encourage you to check out a women-only club. If, on the other hand, you look forward to working out with your spouse or loved one at a coed fitness center, then stay with that option.

Besides, more coed health clubs are partitioning walls and creating special women-only sections. If you seek the best of both fitness worlds, this might be something worth investigating.

Chapter 9

Staying Fit at Work

*B*ack in the old days, when you left for work in the morning, you were guaranteed to be physically exhausted by the end of the day. Work was typically manual labor: walking behind the south end of a horse plowing a row in a northerly direction; carrying the family wash to a nearby stream, where clothes were scrubbed vigorously; hefting bucket after bucket of water from the family well; or chopping firewood to stay warm that night.

Now, humans have become a species of mouse potatoes — a sedentary bunch who spend too many of our waking hours hunched in front of 17-inch computer monitors, staring at pixel-bit screens of digitized information. We perform 3 percent of the physical movements that our great-grandparents did 100 years ago — just 3 percent!

But the corporate world — particularly in the United States and the commerce centers of Europe and Asia — is slowly awakening to the fact that if its workforce is in sorry physical shape, the collective lack of fitness impacts the bottom line. Out-of-shape employees cost companies more in medical premiums (most large corporations are self-insured after a million-dollar threshold is crossed), have higher rates of absenteeism, and are less productive. Duh.

Worker Workouts Work Wonders

Some "early-adapting" corporations such as 3Com, Lucent Technologies, Rodale Press, and Bethlehem Steel have decided that a healthy workforce makes good business sense. They have invested tens of thousands of dollars in fitness equipment and hired trainers to oversee aerobics classes and answer questions about weight-lifting form. The result: healthy, happy employees who work better, smarter, and more effectively for longer periods of time. Those who routinely work out over lunchtime report "thinking clearer" and staying energized throughout the rest of the day — even during those sleep-inducing afternoon meetings formerly marked by droopy eyelids and inattention around the mahogany boardroom table.

In addition, an American College of Sports Medicine study suggests that corporate fitness gyms defuse stress and keep employee injuries and illnesses down. A fitness center on-site is seen as a recruiting tool in today's tight labor market and a cost-effective way to retain employees. Another perk: Having an on-site fitness room saves time for employees who traveled to commercial gyms during their lunch hours.

Given all these benefits of workouts at work, you'd think that a corporate gym is guaranteed in any decent-sized company, but surprisingly, work-site fitness centers remain the province of large businesses and are rarely found in medium- and smaller-sized companies. Dr. Nicholas A. DiNubile, a Philadelphia-area orthopedic surgeon who designs corporate fitness centers and consults with the Philadelphia 76ers, said, "They are not as common as they should be. It really is a wise investment to have an exercising and fit work force. Companies should be developing strategies to activate their workforce. It comes back to them in spades."

Gyms, like companies, come in different sizes

What constitutes a "corporate gym" can range from two aging exercise bikes and a dumbbell set rescued from the local thrift shop to the gleaming $2.7 million WellCom Center at 3Com Inc., in Northern California's Silicon Valley. This 13,500 square-foot facility on 3Com's campus features rows of cycles, treadmills, and weight machines; a hardwood exercise room for aerobics classes; and a sauna where corporate execs can sweat out the previous evening's fat-laden business dinner while they talk shop.

The WellCom Center is open around the clock for 1,800 employees who pay $20 a month, a fraction of what a commercial fitness gym would cost in glitzy Silicon Valley. The membership rolls represent more than 40 percent of the 3Com workforce, and the monthly dues (which pay for upkeep and staffing) ensure that upper management won't close the gym when there's pressure to cut employee amenities.

The only downside to programs such as 3Com's is sustaining employee interest over the long term. The American College of Sports Medicine reports that when a work-site fitness program is first launched, one-third of the employees is likely to join. But half drop out within a few months as good intentions match up against reality. Staying motivated to work out is a far bigger challenge than the physical exertion it takes to exercise your body.

Making the case for a company gym

But what if your company doesn't offer its cherished employees a fitness center? If your company has less than 50 employees, spending budget dollars on a corporate gym probably isn't very cost-effective for management. If you work at a medium-sized or corporate behemoth, however, you definitely have a case to make. Here's how you can get the medicine ball rolling:

1. **Gather the troops.**

   Today's corporate environment features a "top-down" management style, which means that if you're in upper management and would like to see your company open a fitness gym, you can become the self-appointed field general and enlist other VPs and managers in your army.

   If you're among the legions of spear-carriers, however, gather several like-minded colleagues and request a meeting with your manager, who can kick the idea upstairs.

2. **Explain the benefits.**

   Upper management must see in black and white how a corporate fitness center benefits the company as much as it does the rank-and-file employees. Emphasize that employees who work out during the work-day blow off steam, stretch their muscles, and oxygenate their brain cells, all of which makes for sharper workers back in the cubicles. Point out that in a study published by the President's Council on Physical Fitness and Sports, a cost-benefit analysis of corporate gyms found that activity programs saved $1.15 to a whopping $5.52 for every dollar spent. Remind management that they will see productivity gains and that happy employees remain loyal to the company.

3. **Be prepared to cite statistics.**

   Arm yourself with a few statistics from work-site fitness consultant David Spindel:

   - After starting a corporate fitness program, DuPont saw a 47 percent drop in absenteeism over six years.

   - Canadian Life Assurance Co. fitness participants had a 32 percent lower turnover rate than nonparticipants did.

   - At Travelers Corp., the company reduced sick leave by 19 percent among fitness program participants.

4. **Overcome the questions.**

   In today's litigious environment, upper management may express concern over their "exposure" if someone hurts himself while lifting weights in an unsupervised gym. Overcome these objections by working with company attorneys to fashion a liability form for employees to sign before they can use the corporate gym.

Don't be surprised if your manager says that she'll "study" your proposal and promises to "get back" to you. Changes and new ideas take time, but at least you've started the process. In a year or so, you just may have a fitness gym on-site.

Getting the Most from Your Company's Facility

Okay, you've passed all the hurdles, and your company fitness center is open for business. Or you work for a company that already has a gym on-site. How can you maximize your exercise time? Try out these ideas for starters:

✔ **Work out before work.** Morning is the best time to exercise because you can't cancel a completed workout. The workday has a way of taking off, and things that were previously scheduled get put by the wayside. But if you're already done with your workout, you aren't in danger of missing it. Simple logic, but it does make sense. So if you have the time and flexibility in the morning, go for the early workout.

✔ **Work out before or after the lunch hour.** You don't have to be a nerdy tech in MIS to figure out that the busiest time for a corporate gym will be from 12 noon to 1 p.m. and that all the exercise bikes will be taken. Can you flex your schedule? Start lunch at 11:15 a.m.? What about working through your lunch hour and taking your midday break from 1 to 2 p.m.?

✔ **Eat lunch at your desk.** You have a grinder schedule with wall-to-wall meetings all day long. How can you find time to work out, shower, and eat lunch? If your schedule is so tight that you don't have time to work out *and* pass through the employee cafeteria, eat a homemade lunch at your desk while you prepare for your next meeting.

✔ **Work out during rush hour.** City streets, thoroughfares, and freeways are jammed from 5 to 6 p.m. Stay away from the maddening crowd and work out at the end of the business day. Rather than waste precious time sitting in traffic, maximize your time by sitting on an exercise cycle and burning off calories. Let the freeways thin out before you drive home.

What to Do If Your Company Doesn't Have a Fitness Room

Corporate fitness centers are catching on with more and more large companies. A nationwide survey by William M. Mercer, Inc., a consulting firm based in New York, found that 41 percent of companies with 750 employees or more had fitness facilities. But that leaves 59 percent of large companies with *no* corporate gyms, and the percentage is undoubtedly higher for smaller firms. If your place of employment doesn't have a workout facility, I can think of plenty of small ways that you can exercise during your workday:

- **Park in the far end of the employee parking lot and walk to your office.** The time it takes to look for a parking spot near the front door can be better spent hoofing it from the outer reaches.

- **Take the stairs every chance you can.** Climbing stairs is great aerobic activity. Why take an elevator, especially if you're only traveling a couple of floors to the next meeting? (See the "Stairway to heaven" sidebar in this chapter.)

- **Go to a nearby fitness club on your lunch hour.** Working out at noon-time gives you a lesser chance to "bag it" at the end of the day. You may be able to get your company to pay for the monthly dues, or you may find that the fitness club offers a special group rate to your company.

- **Engage in your physical activity after work.** If you just don't have time to drive to a fitness center, work out, shower, and eat in one hour (which is understandable), then get your exercise after work. Take the time to play tennis, go on a long walk with a friend, participate in a basketball league, go swimming at the local Y, or push plates at your local gym.

Wear comfortable sneakers or walking shoes to work and carry a pair of your work shoes in a bag (or store a pair at your desk). You can slip on your sneakers when you have to walk to another building, go for a break-time walk, or make a mini-trek during lunchtime. Bringing a second pair of shoes to work is a hassle, but with a little effort, you can make big health strides.

Stairway to heaven

In this "I've got no time to exercise" age, there's a great exercise alternative just steps away at your place of work: the stairwell. Lifting your body one step at a time is a great exercise for your heart, muscles, and bones. Taking the stairs is easy to do and can be accomplished while wearing a suit, tie, and wingtips (or "corporate casual"). You don't get sweaty, and you don't need an appointment.

Small amounts of physical activity throughout the day can provide significant health benefits, and for many white-collar workers, the stairwell is the *only* way to snatch some quick aerobic exercise. A Harvard Alumni Health Study of 11,000 men found that those who climbed at least 20 floors per week had a 20 percent lower risk of stroke and of death from all causes during the study period. Twenty floors per week isn't much, folks: that's only four flights of stairs a day. Put your mind to this corporate form of step aerobics, and you may end up climbing 20 floors per day!

So why doesn't everyone automatically take the stairs? Given the choice between using the elevator and an adjacent flight of stairs, people vote with their feet, leading them straight into the elevator. Researchers from Johns Hopkins University Medical Center in Baltimore observed that 95 percent of people rode the elevator instead of taking the stairway. Many people, while concentrating on the next task or where they're going, flat out forget to take the stairs.

Kelly Brownell, a Yale University obesity expert, contends that we live in a "toxic physical activity environment," where automobiles, elevators, moving walkways, automatic doors, and TV remote controls make it too darn easy to go through life without moving one more muscle than necessary.

She's probably right, but here's a way to break through the barriers of automation: Ask your company to erect reminders of staircase exercise — signs next to the elevator that say "Be fit: Take the stairs" or "Why *weight* for the elevator?"

What if your floor is ten stories up? You can take the elevator halfway there and then disembark and walk. Within a few days, you'll be able to climb six floors and then eight floors and then all ten floors in a snap.

Keep this thought in mind as you huff and puff while negotiating the stairwell during the day: Not only is taking the stairs a free fitness opportunity, but you're being *paid* to exercise as you're walking on company time!

Chapter 10

Home Sweet Gym: Buying Exercise Equipment

*H*ome exercise equipment is hot and sure to get hotter as people experience the benefits of state-of-the art treadmills, stair steppers, and gyms *zu Hause* (in the home), available any time of the day or night. The price of fitness equipment — like computers — continues to go down each year, but the quality gets better and better. The convenience of home fitness machines can be liberating, as long as you use the stuff.

You could say that we're fans of home exercise equipment, judging by the number of pieces we keep in our Orlando home. Our game room is home to a Precor 9.4SP treadmill that has more miles on the odometer than half the rental cars in the Disney World parking lot. The treadmill allows me to work up a sweat on those days when I have don't have a tennis game or when a sudden thunderstorm sweeps through Central Florida.

We park a Lifestep 9500 stair stepper in the guest room, where I've noticed some of our houseguests pumping away. Sticking out like a sore thumb in our TV room, however, is a Lifecycle 9500HR stationary bike — a rusting contraption that's piling up layers of dust and no mileage these days. But I religiously use our StretchMate, a spider-like stretching device that graces a corner of our master bedroom (see Chapter 15). I often stretch for five to ten minutes before retiring. That's all you need.

Choosing to Bring It Home

Home exercise equipment works fine for most people, but it has to make financial and fitness sense before you invest hard-earned money and valuable time. You should consider purchasing fitness equipment if you fall into these categories:

- You have a hectic work schedule that doesn't allow you enough breathing room to work out during the day.

- You can't leave the kids home alone while you work out away from the house.

- You want to do some cross-training. You may enjoy playing tennis three times a week for exercise but recognize the need to lift weights at home.

- You live more than 15 minutes from a fitness club. Remember, if the time cost is too high, you probably won't travel to a club to work out.

- You don't want to pay hefty monthly membership fees or be locked into yearly contracts at a trendy gym.

- You prefer not to be ogled by sweaty Neanderthals working up a lather on the stair stepper next to you.

- You fear that curvaceous young women in their skimpy aerobics outfits could be hazardous to your health — especially if your wife catches you looking at them.

- You don't want to show your not-ready-for-prime-time legs to the world.

Sales of exercise equipment to people between the ages of 45 and 64 rose 53 percent in 1998 alone. One of the selling points of home exercise equipment is that the cost of financing the equipment is about what you would pay in monthly dues at a nice club.

As a general rule, you will pay around $40 a month for three years to finance $1,000 worth of equipment, so if you purchase a True treadmill, Body Guard stair climber, and dumbbell set for $2,000, you'll be paying about $80 a month for three years. After 36 payments, you own the equipment. I don't want to throw a wet blanket over financing home exercise equipment, but I must point out that most financing plans charge 19 percent interest, which means a $2,000 purchase will end up costing you $2,700 on equipment that loses half its value in three years. If you're going to buy new, I recommend that you pay cash or put it on your credit card (if you pay your statement in full each month).

You should carefully think through the purchase of home exercise equipment because after the machine is in your home, it could be there for a *long* time. The cost of changing your mind and returning equipment is steep — you'll be docked for restocking and shipping fees, in most cases. Fitness equipment that's a few years old can be a notoriously tough sell, which explains why you see so many cheap exercise bikes lined up at your neighborhood Disabled American Veterans thrift shop.

I issue this warning because some people experience buyer's remorse after the UPS man has lugged several heavy boxes to the front door and said, "Sign here." What begins as a promise ("I'm going to use this every day") too often turns into a host of lamentations ("When am I going to find time?" or "How am I going to pay this off?"). That's because the first thing people drop from their busy schedules is exercise, and staying motivated requires almost as much work as working out. You can count on your interest in using home exercise equipment waning after a "honeymoon" period. You don't want to allow two months to pass before noticing that you haven't worked out at all.

I'm not trying to cast a negative light on home exercise equipment, however, because high-quality machines can be a superb addition to your fitness regimen — just what the doctor ordered in many cases. Home fitness equipment can also augment a "lite" physical regimen of walking or bike riding for those of you trying to get back in shape after years of inactivity.

Taking It One Step at a Time

If you're serious about exploring the home gym option, you need to walk yourself through these five steps:

Identify your fitness needs and then educate yourself

First and foremost, home exercise equipment should fit your long-term fitness goals. (See Chapter 7 to find out which equipment, if any, is for you.) And if an apparatus is going to gobble up space in your den or bedroom, you may want to make sure that it is easy and fun to use, or it will eventually end up as an elaborate home for wayward insects or clothes.

Another thing to consider is whether you want to replicate an outdoor activity in the safety and comfort of your home. You may like riding a bike for exercise, which means an indoor cycle complements that activity. If you enjoy striding like a cross-country skier, you should consider a ski simulator machine. A ski simulator wouldn't be a good fit for me because I didn't grow up in snow country.

To find out what type of machine you're looking for, you have to educate yourself. You begin by inviting personal trainers for their recommendations, talking to sales staff at specialty fitness stores, asking friends to describe their experiences, and reading up on the latest developments in home exercise equipment on the Internet and in fitness periodicals.

Choose a budget

Although many specialty fitness stores have financing plans, you're best off paying cash because you will save money in the long run. If you decide that $500 is your limit and all the new stuff is a thousand bucks or more, you'll have to venture into the used-equipment market. Ask yourself this question: "Should I buy good-quality used equipment or lesser-quality new equipment?" Your answer should be a slam dunk. Always purchase quality over newness.

Shop around

For the moment, I'll assume that you have the money to buy new. This is where it pays to be a good shopper. Drop by a specialty fitness store and ask questions. Sales people understand that customers do not make purchases on the first visit, so they are used to "tire kickers."

Then you can drop by a bookstore and purchase several fitness magazines. Study the advertisements for home exercise machines. Drive to your local library, and page through back issues of *Consumer Reports, Consumers Digest,* and other consumer-related magazines for their recommendations. If you are in the market for a treadmill, look at the advertisements found in walking and running magazines. Want an exercise bike? Read the ads found in cycling magazines.

The next step is to turn to the Internet and type **exercise machines** into your favorite search engine. A couple of informative Web sites are thefitnessoutlet.com and ifit.com. The *Consumer Reports* Web site (www.consumerreports.org) allows you access to its archives for $3.95 per every 30 days of access. Keep in mind, however, that *Consumer Reports* reviews machines sold by mass-market retailers and leaves out many of the brands sold by specialty fitness stores. The machines rated a "Best Buy" contain quality construction and good features at a competitive price, but the capability of these machines to provide an above-average workout is not heavily weighted. *Consumer Reports'* buying guidelines, however, will give you a good overview of the types of home exercise equipment on the market and a list of features to help you ask the right questions.

You can often trust a friend's recommendations. Ask what she likes and dislikes about her home exercise equipment, where she purchased the equipment, whether it was a good deal, what financing plans the store offered, and whether the sales staff treated her fairly. Continue to network. Word-of-mouth really counts.

You will find stores selling home exercise equipment listed under "Exercise" in the Yellow Pages. Start with specialty fitness retailers that offer a variety of new, pre-owned, and refurbished equipment. These stores are usually staffed by knowledgeable sales people, as opposed to department store or sporting goods warehouses where the inexperienced sales staff tends not to be educated in the products and physical fitness in general.

Determine what fits in your home

You won't know what you have room for until you find out how big each machine's "footprint" is and measure the nook or cranny into which you're thinking about plopping your machine. After you make the space measurements, add another 15 percent just to be sure. Don't forget to consider ceiling height — some multistation machines stand 11 feet tall — and the logistics of getting the machine into your house. Unless you've arranged for delivery, you may have trouble getting that new treadmill up to the second floor.

You may consider these possible places for your home exercise equipment:

- Spare bedroom
- Family room
- Loft
- Patio
- Sewing room
- Home office
- Garage
- Attic

Take a closer look at these options.

The patio is a no-no; the outdoor elements will ruin your investment faster than you can say "Jack Frost."

The garage could work if you live in a temperate climate, but most times of the year, it's too hot or too cold to exercise in the garage.

How much room will my machine take up?

You may find helpful these general guidelines on how much room you'll need for different types of in-home exercise equipment. Of course, these numbers are approximate and depend on the particular model that you purchase:

- ✔ Treadmill: 20 square feet
- ✔ Bike: 7 to 15 square feet
- ✔ Stair climber: 10-20 square feet
- ✔ Rowing machine: 12-14 square feet
- ✔ Single-station gym: 20-40 square feet

- ✔ Multistation gym: 50-100 square feet
- ✔ Free weights: 20-50 square feet
- ✔ Ski machine: 20-25 square feet

Don't forget that many of the new treadmills fold up when you're finished, which saves space when you're not using the machine. And remember to consider the shape of the equipment; you need 15 square feet for some bikes, but none will fit in a 1-by-15-foot space.

Ditto for an attic, unless it has plenty of circulation and comfortable temperatures throughout the year. Trust me: If the temperature is too hot or cold, you won't exercise. For those living in warm locales, be sure that you can place the machine near an air conditioner or fan. You will appreciate cool air blowing across your face.

The best options are a spare bedroom, home office, sewing room, loft, or den. I don't recommend the family room because exercise machines make lots of noise, and you'll disturb others. Your spouse may not want a noisy treadmill messing up the family room. Try to find some free square footage in a more isolated area of the house, especially if you plan on using your equipment at odd hours — for example, at 6 a.m. while most of the family is still asleep.

Speaking of noise, apartments and home exercise equipment don't mix very well. Apartments are famous for paper-thin walls that allow you to listen to your neighbor's arguments or squeaky bed frame. If you think you're going to fire up your rowing machine at 5:45 a.m. and not have your neighbor notice, you should think again. You may either have to exercise between the hours of 8 a.m. and 8 p.m. or wait until you move into your own single-family detached home.

Put the machine where you have the best chance to use it. In other words, if your treadmill has to be within earshot of a television (or you'll go stir crazy), you must place it in a room where you have a television set. If you don't have another room with a TV, go buy an inexpensive model. I enjoy watching ESPN's *SportsCenter*, a little CNN news, a History Channel program — I can usually find something halfway worthwhile to land on. You'll find a second or third TV to be a cheap price to remain motivated.

Very few people can churn their legs on a treadmill or pump an exercise bike without some type of outside stimulus. Otherwise, it's like watching paint dry while you pump away. I have always needed something to help pass the time. When I jog or use the treadmill, I listen to audiotapes of fascinating and interesting speakers or audiobooks. Accomplishing two tasks at once allows me to "redeem" the time.

Finally, you can always read while you work out. (You're welcome to read this book, too.) Reading works best for exercise bikes, because only your legs are pumping and your upper body remains quiet. I find it hard to stride on a treadmill or pump a stair stepper and still read at the same time — I'm just bouncing around too much.

Try out the equipment

Just as you wouldn't purchase a car without a test drive, you shouldn't purchase any home exercise equipment without an audition. You can test equipment at one or more of the following places:

- **At a friend's house.** Call up a friend and ask if you can come over to try her fitness equipment. Ask her whether she's had any trouble with the machine, if the equipment has been easy to learn how to use, and if it is noisy or disruptive. Watch out, however. She may try to sell her used machine to you! (Just joking.)

- **At your fitness center.** You should already be familiar with the cardio-vascular equipment at your health club. If your gym carries Schwinn Airdyne dual-action bikes and you think the same model or some other home exercise bike would be great to have for those days when you can't get to the gym, ask the staff members for their recommendations.

- **At fitness equipment retailers.** Stores that specialize in fitness equipment have a showroom of new and used equipment for you to try. You should shop in shorts and a polo shirt so you can try the machine in as close to "live" conditions as possible.

- **At sporting goods stores.** Amidst the mountains of sneakers, clothes, and accessories such as bats, rackets, and clubs, you will find a home fitness section. Because sporting goods stores sell everything under the sun, the staff's knowledge of specialty fitness equipment is a mile wide and an inch deep. The quality of the fitness equipment does not match what you can find in specialty stores. Mass-market retailers are willing to let slow-moving merchandise leave the sales floor at a significant discount, however, during their periodic "sales." The best times to shop for fitness equipment are the spring (after the slowdown in New Year's resolution shoppers) and summer (when busy families are vacationing or demand has dropped because many people are pursuing outdoor activities). You should also shop in workout clothes so you can give the equipment a try.

✔ **At garage sales.** A lot of used fitness equipment gets unloaded at garage sales. Because the first rule with garage sales is *caveat emptor* ("Let the buyer beware"), your exercise machine comes with no guarantee. Ask for a demonstration of the machine. Then try it yourself, making sure you ask questions. Plug in the electrical cord to make sure that all the features work. Expect the quality of home exercise equipment to be spotty at garage sales because that's the nature of the beast. Final reminder: Many times, you're buying discontinued models, which means parts are either no longer available or hard to come by.

✔ **At the homes of private sellers.** You've scoured the classified ads, and now you're making the rounds. Buying used from a private party can be an excellent avenue — *if you're an educated buyer.* The high-quality machines sell quickly, but you don't find many excellent, low-mileage machines for sale because most people are happy to keep them around. What you see being sold in most newspapers is a lot of junk — just like in garage sales. Be sure to try before you buy; you'll get a good idea of how the machine sounds and fits in a living environment.

The other downside to buying through newspaper ads is the time it takes to call, learn whether the machine is worth viewing, and drive to the person's home. If you choose to go to this much trouble, then take cash. Not only are private parties very reluctant to take checks, but cash talks and you-know-what walks. Sometimes a wad of bills can make your lowball offer irresistible to someone desperate to get that exercise bike off his hands.

Danger, Will Robinson! A Word about Infomercials

Glistening models and leather-skinned actors may make a "Millennium Home Gym" look like the greatest deal since the Louisiana Purchase, but I would not recommend buying any exercise equipment from an infomercial. These 30-minute staged and choreographed presentations are designed to manipulate your emotions into making a spontaneous purchase. Infomercials present "experts" who breathlessly reveal their latest "research" about the product. Infomercials constantly cut in testimonial sound bites from average Joes and Joelles who claim that their lives were changed after using some "bun trainer" for 30 days. Infomercials assert that their uniquely designed movements provide "better workouts" in "less time." If only any of this hokum were true. You're being hyped. Zap the channel!

Besides, you can't test the equipment before purchasing, with good reason. If you test-drove some of this junk, you'd never agree to buy it. Yes, many infomercials offer a money-back guarantee, but the tiny print also states that you're responsible for disassembling the exercise machine and paying the shipping costs to return 200 pounds of plastic, rubber, and metal to the manufacturer. The freight bill can range from $50 to $200.

The last time I checked, more than 60 home exercise equipment infomercials pop up on late-night "indie" stations and cable channels. From my quick perusal, anything for abs (short for abdominal stomach muscles) is *hot*. As the camera focuses on a body builder's midsection, you are told that you can have the same killer, chiseled, washboard, twisted-steel, rock-hard abs if only you'll purchase this latest ab breakthrough. Why, for prices ranging from $39.95, plus shipping and handling, to $119.80, you can purchase any of the following:

- ✔ Ab Rocker
- ✔ Ab Sculptor
- ✔ Abslide
- ✔ Ab Trainer
- ✔ Ab Twister
- ✔ Ab Works

I hate to break the bad news to you, but you're not going to get killer abs in 30 days. You'd have to do crunches around the clock for several years before you'd even approach the look of those rock-hard abs modeled on TV.

Infomercials are a bad bet and practically guarantee you that you'll pay an inflated price to compensate for the expensive marketing and celebrity endorsements. Celebs can move product, however, which proves that P.T. Barnum's dictum still reigns.

What to Know Before You Buy

You can pay princely prices for fresh-out-of-the-box, state-of-the-art, decked-out-with-gizmos fitness equipment, or pauper sums for yesterday's equipment, which may or may not have been state-of-the-art when it hit the marketplace. This section is a rundown of what new and used equipment costs, plus comments regarding several salient features. (See Chapter 7 for details on the fitness benefits that exercise machines provide.)

When you're buying new

Make no mistake: The latest generation of fitness machines is better constructed and more effective than ever. You have more options at your fingertips — features that allow you to create customized programs that change the speed, intensity, and resistance to exactly what you want. If you're planning on making your home into a personal fitness shrine, you won't go wrong by buying new — as long as you make an informed choice.

Treadmills

Selling point: If you're going to buy only one piece of home fitness equipment, make it a treadmill. Treadmills allow for walking or jogging on a smooth surface in the comfort of your home, surrounded by your favorite media (television, CD player, or reading material). New treadmills come with five-year warranties on parts and one- to two-year warranties that cover parts *and* labor.

Features: Electronic models offer a variety of speeds to "move" you along. Higher-quality treadmills can change incline and monitor heart rate and calories burned. Your treadmill should have a continuous-duty horsepower rating of at least 2.0 hp. (Continuous duty indicates the power of the machine use after use, day after day. "Peak" horsepower is a meaningless term used to sell inferior equipment.) Control panels — which display speed, incline, distance, time, and heart rate — come in LCD (liquid crystal display) and LED (light emitting diode), the latter being more expensive.

Brands to look for: True, Landice, and Precor

What you can expect to pay: Plan to spend $1,000 and up for a quality treadmill, with high-end treadmills averaging $3,000.

Downside: None, except for the expense.

Stationary bikes

Selling point: These popular exercise machines have been around for decades and are getting better and more dependable all the time. Easy to use, even while watching TV or reading, stationary bikes provide non-impact aerobic exercise for the lower body in a hurry.

Features: Exercise bikes come in three different models: upright, recumbent, and dual-action. (See Chapter 7 for descriptions.)

Brands to look for: Schwinn and Body Guard.

What you can expect to pay: You can find decent stationary bicycles for $500, but for a couple hundred dollars more, you can purchase a recumbent model or a dual-action bike that allows you to work your upper arms while you pedal. Quality and features pick up when you cross the $1,000 threshold. You can spend more than $2,000 for sophisticated models.

Downside: You might get saddle sore pedaling for a long time, but that's not much of a downside.

Strength-training machines

Selling point: You have the ability to isolate specific upper and lower body muscle groups while you perform anaerobic (or strength-training) exercise.

Features: Chest and shoulder press machines, leg press, and extension machines provide a well-rounded workout.

Brands to look for: Hoist, Schwinn, and Parabody.

What you can expect to pay: An entry-level machine costs about $1,000, but you can expect to pay between $2,000 and $3,000 for an excellent multistation machine.

Downside: A quality home gym is not cheap and must be assembled by a professional. A multistation machine is a space-grabber and not easily moved.

Elliptical machines

Selling point: They are new and hot, and they give you a total body workout with no learning curve, so put your feet in the foot pedals and go!

Features: These machines are a cross between walking, bicycling, and stepping, but you also receive a modest upper-body workout while you pump handlebars that move in sync with your feet.

Brands to look for: Schwinn.

What you can expect to pay: Around $1,000.

Downside: Some say elliptical machines are too easy, while others feel they are too intense. You either swear by them or swear at them.

Rowing machines

Selling point: The cadence of rowing is appealing to certain people.

Features: Seats should be sturdy as you push and pull your body.

Brands to look for: Schwinn.

What you can expect to pay: Around $1,000 for a decent machine.

Downside: Rowing is not an easy exercise, especially for those in their middle-age years. Rowers are not recommended for those with back problems.

Stair steppers

Selling point: You work up a sweat quickly and feel the burn in the thighs.

Features: Look for step machines that are "independently linked," meaning that the footpads move independently of each other. "Dependent linked" machines (when one foot pad moves forward, the other automatically moves backward) are awkward to use and cheaply made.

Brands to look for: StairMaster, Body Guard, and Schwinn.

When you're ready to make a purchase

You've done your homework. You've visited the retailer once or twice to narrow down your choices. These do's and don'ts help you when you're a "today" buyer for home exercise equipment:

✔ **Don't skimp on basic features.** Each machine has different features that you shouldn't live without. Find out what they are.

✔ **Do give it a real test.** Almost any treadmill feels great for 3 minutes, but you have to walk on a machine for 20 minutes to determine whether it vibrates excessively or makes lots of noise. For multipurpose weight machines, do a set of 10 repetitions.

✔ **Don't buy the bells and whistles.** Do you really need an LED (light emitting diode) display on your new treadmill? Probably not.

✔ **Do check out the top-of-the-line equipment.** Like anything else, you get what you pay for. Buy the best name-brand equipment that you can afford because you're going to have it for a while.

✔ **Do have an open mind.** Yes, treadmills are popular and reliable, but elliptical trainers also provide functional movement. Maybe you're the type who likes dual-action exercise bikes.

✔ **Don't believe everything you hear.** You'll hear lots of claims, lots of bad-mouthing of other products, and lots of hot air. Talk to as many people as you can to form a consensus.

✔ **Do ask about the warranty and repair programs.** Top fitness equipment retailers gain their reputation in customer service.

✔ **Do look for the "Made in USA" tag.** The imports have yet to catch up to the quality of American-made fitness equipment.

✔ **Don't buy the first thing you see.** You only get to make a major purchase once. Avoid expensive mistakes.

✔ **Do take your spouse or partner with you when shopping.** Two minds are better than one, right?

What you can expect to pay: You'll find machines in all prices ranges. Top-of-the-line stair steppers run between $1,500 to $2,500.

Downside: Low-quality steppers make you never want to step on a machine again. Choose a stair stepper with smooth motion.

Dumbbells

Selling point: Dumbbells are an inexpensive complement to aerobic exercise. You buy only as many dumbbells as you think you need.

Brands to look for: None in particular.

What you can expect to pay: Chrome or hex dumbbells range from 50 cents to $2 a pound. Most people can get away for around $50 total.

Downside: None. Dumbbells are dumbbells.

When you're buying used

A couple of things to keep in mind when buying used fitness equipment. First, the warranties are not transferable, so you are on your own in that department. Second, you will have to transport the piece of equipment to your home. Can you borrow a friend's truck? You may have to disassemble and then reassemble the fitness machine to get it into your house. Is that something you're capable of doing?

Quality fitness equipment generally holds half its value in the first two to three years. In other words, if a stationary bike cost $1,000, you should expect to pay $500 for a two-year-old model. Equipment older than five years is generally worth 20 percent of its original value.

Treadmills

What to look for: Up until a couple of years ago, treadmills came in non-motorized versions, which meant you had to do all the work to keep the belt moving. Don't buy a used non-motorized treadmill, which is bad for your back. Look for a motorized one with at least a 2.0 hp motor.

The used machine market: Between $250 and $500.

Stationary bikes

What to look for: Individuals with knee, hip, and ankle problems generally find the upright bikes to be more comfortable. Individuals with abdominal or back problems prefer recumbent exercise bikes, which tend to be more expensive than their upright counterparts.

The used machine market: $100 to $500.

If you buy from the Internet

Suppose that you walk into your neighborhood specialty fitness outlet and do some shopping. You decide that a Landice treadmill is the one for you. The price: $2,500. *Whoa, that's a bunch of money*, you say. *And all that sales tax.*

So you go home and get on the Internet. A few clicks, and you find a "retailer" in Wisconsin who will sell you the exact same Landice model for $250 less — and no sales tax. "I want it," you say.

Not a good idea, and let me tell you why. If you ever have any problems with your Landice treadmill, you're not going to be able to go to your local dealer. He services only what he sells. The vendor in Wisconsin won't know whom to call in your hometown. The manufacturer is caught in the middle but can't force his local dealer to help you.

Yes, you paid less, but part of your "win" was eaten by extra shipping costs — $150 in this case. If you decide that this isn't the exercise bike of your dreams and you want to return it, the fine print says that the Wisconsin dealer can charge you a 20 percent "restocking fee." Oops. There goes $425, and you still have to pay $100 to ship the heavy son-of-gun to points north. That's true even if your equipment arrives in a scratch-and-dent condition from the shipper.

The Internet is a great tool to purchase books and airline tickets, but not exercise equipment.

Strength-training machines

What to look for: Quality weight-stack machines are made of tubular steel and come with lateral pull-down attachments, squat attachments, curl bars, and weight-stack guards.

The used machine market: $500 to $2,000.

Elliptical machines

What to look for: Because elliptical machines are just a few years old, don't purchase any "first generation" machines. Manufacturers worked out the bugs for the newer models.

The used machine market: $250 to $750.

Rowing machines

What to look for: A machine that still functions well.

The used machine market: $100 to $500.

You'll find a home gym for every budget

If you're going to bring fitness home, you can spend a little money or a *lot* of money. Here you'll find three options, but feel free to mix 'n' match according to your spending mood.

The "Price Is No Object" Home Gym

- Hoist multistation, four-weight stack weight-resistance machine (cost: $6,000)

- Top-of-the-line True treadmill (cost: $5,000)

- "Virtual reality" cycle with a video screen and wheels that bank to simulate the hills and curves of mountain biking (cost: $6,000)

- Body Guard stationary bike (cost: $2,000)

- Full rack of chrome-plated dumbbells (cost: $1,250)

- 33-inch flat-screen TV (cost: $1,500)

- CD sound system (cost: $1,000)

- Cardiosport heart monitor (cost: $180)

Total cost: $22,930

The "Be Reasonable" Gym

- Schwinn treadmill (cost: $2,000)

- Schwinn multistation gym with one weight stack (cost: $2,000)

- Set of hex dumbbells (cost: $300)

- Adequate sound system (cost: $500)

Total cost: $5,300

The Budget Home Gym

- Used exercise bike purchased from a private party (cost: $250)

- CD boom box (cost: $39)

- Several garage sale dumbbells (cost: $5)

Total cost: $294

Possible Accessories for Any Gym

- Mat to catch the rivulets of sweat that drip off your body and minimize carpet marks

- Stretching mat for warm-ups and cool down

- Eight-foot long wooden bar for stretching, mounted on a wall

- Heart monitor

- Reading rack for your cardiovascular machine so you can catch up on your reading while working your heart

- Mini-refrigerator stocked with Evian, Gatorade, and herbal ice teas

Ski-simulator machines

What to look for: If you're a die-hard cross-country skier, then you may be in the market for a NordicTrack machine or some other brand of ski simulator. The legs push wooden ski-like rails against resistance while the arms pump a pulley in a way that simulates the skiing arm movement.

The used machine market: $50 to $200. Careful. It can be difficult repairing or finding parts for NordicTrack machines.

Stair steppers

What to look for: You want a step machine with independent leg action.

The used machine market: $100 to $500.

Dumbbells

What to look for: Some people prefer hexagon-shaped dumbbells because they won't roll when you place them on the ground.

The used dumbbell market: Dumbbells aren't a high-demand item, so they don't have much resale value. If you see a set at a garage sale, bargain hard!

Gyms on Wheels: Fitness Delivered to Your Door

One way to work out at home without purchasing any equipment or finding room to store the stuff is to employ a "gym-on-wheels" company that pulls into your driveway at a time that works best for you. Just call it "takeout fitness" because you can order a workout much like a Domino's deep-dish pizza.

Using such names as Fitness to You, Wellness on Wheels and Exercise Express, these mobile fitness entrepreneurs outfit a 20-foot van or small RV with steppers, bikes, treadmills, strength-training equipment, and a CD stereo system. A driver/personal trainer steers the fitness van to your driveway or sidewalk at the appointed time, and voilà, you have a well-equipped mini gym just steps from your front door.

You also have the services of a personal trainer to direct your workout, which lasts for 30, 45, or 60 minutes, depending on the length of your appointment. The trainer will put you through the paces of chest and shoulder press machines, leg press and extension machines, a series of dumbbells, and back-strengthening stretches — all to the beat of your favorite fast-paced music blaring from the Bose speakers.

You may be asking yourself: Why would I want to work out in a glorified truck? Convenience is the biggest reason. If you're in the midst of a demanding career in which every 30 minutes is a luxurious commodity, then a fitness-on-wheels program may be just what you need. Most clients are busy executives, according to those in the business. Takeout fitness is an excellent avenue for those rehabbing from sports injuries. If your doctor has ordered rehabilitation following an injury but you find getting to a rehab facility is just too difficult — or painful — consider fitness-to-go. You won't have to wait your turn at a crowded rehabilitation facility.

The benefits of mobile fitness vans

These are the many upsides of having a fitness van come to your home:

- **Motivation:** If you have trouble staying motivated, the sight of a mobile fitness van pulling into your driveway would be a tangible reminder that you're going to work out — and you'd better be ready! You can run but you can't hide from your appointment. Besides, cancellation fees run 100 percent, so you're going to have to pay for the workout even if you decide to close the curtains and not answer the doorbell.

- **Time:** The mobile gym comes at the time that works best for you. If you're the type who needs to put something in a DayTimer to get it done, then the discipline of keeping a fitness appointment will work for you. If your schedule is so tight that the only way you could work out is if the fitness center comes to you, then consider making an appointment.

- **Having a personal trainer:** Some of us would never splurge on a personal trainer at a brick-and-mortar gym, but because a fitness van comes with a PT, we can justify the added expense. Personal trainers can exhort you to new fitness levels and tailor the right fitness program for you.

- **Focus:** A personal trainer can't do the workout for you, but he sure can keep you on task.

- **Intensity:** Because you know your time is limited, you can do your half-hour or one-hour workout intensely and without waiting for various machines to open up.

- **Freedom of choice:** You don't like the personal trainer? Have the company send someone else. Don't like the setup of the fitness van? Try another fitness-on-wheels company. You remain in the driver's seat. Contrast your freedom of choice with locked-in, yearlong contracts at your neighborhood fitness center.

- **Privacy:** Those sensitive to "body issues" or their weight will find the privacy of a mobile fitness van liberating. It's like working out with a trainer in the privacy of your own home with equipment you'd find in a well-maintained gym.

- **Music preferences:** Tired of hearing "classic rock" music — or, worse, rap music — at your local gym? You control the sounds emanating from the stereo speakers. Choose your own motivating music and never wear a portable cassette player again.

The drawbacks of "fitness to go"

You will pay a premium for the convenience and personalization of mobile fitness visits. Most companies charge $60 and up for a visit — a cost comparable to most gyms' personal trainers. But it may be well worth the investment to you.

Another problem is that because takeout fitness is so new, not every city has a mobile gym service. Check "Exercise & Physical Fitness Programs" in your Yellow Pages, on the Internet, or at an "announcement board" at your local gym. You can also ask around.

Part III
Exercising for Life

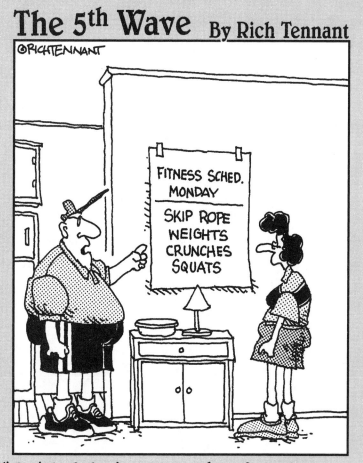

The 5th Wave By Rich Tennant

FITNESS SCHED.
MONDAY

SKIP ROPE
WEIGHTS
CRUNCHES
SQUATS

"I AM following the schedule! Today
I skipped the rope, then I skipped
the weights, then I skipped the crunches..."

In this part . . .

This part starts by covering some of the building blocks of a good workout: a good night's sleep, comfortable clothing, and good shoes. A whole chapter is devoted to feet because if the feet ain't happy, ain't nobody happy.

Once you're dressed properly from head to toe, you're ready for some gym work. This part leads you step-by-step through warm-up exercises, stretching movements, upper-body exercise routines, and lower-body exercise routines — complete with dozens of photographs. You'll learn that when your workout is over, you need to cool down with light exercise for several minutes and replenish your lost bodily fluids. You'll drink up the information on water and sports beverages such as Gatorade.

Chapter 11

First Things First: Getting a Good Night's Sleep

S leep is a basic necessity of life, something as fundamental to your health as air, food, and water. When you sleep well, you wake up feeling refreshed, revitalized — and ready to exercise. "Sleep plays a major role in preparing the body and brain for an alert, productive, psychologically, and physiologically healthy tomorrow," said Dr. James B. Maas, author of *Power Sleep*.

When it comes to exercise and sleep, however, it's a chicken-or-egg question: Which comes first? Does sleeping longer give you more energy to exercise? Or does a well-rounded exercise program cause you to sleep better? I believe that the answer is the former. Plenty of rest rejuvenates the body, makes us eager to attack the following day with energetic gusto, and may be viewed as a major component of fitness. You are less vulnerable to illness, getting in accidents, or becoming depressed.

On the flip side, I concede that working out also prepares us for falling asleep. I always felt that being physically tired — that good, bone-tired feeling I had when I trained hard that day — resulted in deep, restful sleep. I experienced no problems getting plenty of sleep when I played on the WTA (Women's Tennis Association) tour. (I admit that playing the professional tennis circuit was not the same as waking up at 6:15 a.m. to catch a subway into the city.) Like most of my contemporaries on the pro tour, I usually slept nine or ten hours a night. (I know — you'd give anything to be able to sleep nine hours!) As a young mom, I value sleep more than ever these days. My goal continues to be eight hours of sleep each night.

Waking Up to the Importance of Sleep

Allow me to issue a wake-up call about the importance of sleep: I believe that fitness-conscious people have overlooked sleep as an important part of their regimen. It's a fact: A good night's sleep revitalizes tired bodies, gives us more energy, and helps us think more clearly throughout the day. If you're going to take fitness seriously, you should try to sleep at least eight hours a night — or at least 30 to 60 minutes more a night than you are sleeping currently. When you're well rested, you're less likely to cancel a workout. Your attitude is going to be better because you don't feel as tired. Your muscles are going to be properly rested.

Statistics tell us that the typical American suffers from a "sleep gap" or the lack of a good night's sleep. American adults sleep an average of only seven hours a night; this number is down 20 percent from a century ago when American adults slept an average of nine hours a night, according to the National Sleep Foundation. Although Americans sleep an average of only seven hours a night, 98 percent think that sleep is important to good health — as important as nutrition and exercise, said a National Sleep Foundation survey from 1998.

If you only knew how unhealthy this lack-of-sleep trend is! Well, I'm going to tell you. Researchers from the University of Chicago's Department of Medicine found that insufficient rest makes you old before your time. The University of Chicago researchers restricted the sleeping hours of 11 healthy men — ages 18 to 27 — to four hours a night for six days. The sleep-deprived men began experiencing metabolic and hormonal changes usually found in people over 60 years of age. In other words, their sleep debt hurt their ability to metabolize carbohydrates (sugars and starches) and produce gland secretions. (The test subjects reversed those trends within one week by sleeping 12 hours each night.)

You may realize that you are not getting enough sleep, but you're not doing anything about it. I think I can point the finger at one of the thieves of your sleep time — the television. Americans watch, on average, four hours of television per day, and the television is on in the background for another four hours a day, reported Harvard researchers David Campbell, Steven Yonish, and Robert Putnam in 1999. Because you probably don't get home until the early evening, this fact means that your television is on from the time you step inside the front door until "lights out." You always seem to watch one more program, one more *20/20* segment, one more news story, and before you know it, the time is way past 11 p.m.

You may say that TV is the least necessary part of your life, yet you may devote more of your free time to watching television than any other leisure activity. This trend must change! Trade the TV time for exercise time, and you'll never regret it.

Super Snoozing in Six Steps

If you receive less than eight delicious hours of sleep each night, here are some ways you may increase your deposits in your sleep bank:

1. **Find out how much sleep you need.** On your next vacation, go to bed when you feel tired, but don't set an alarm. Sleep as long as you can — until you're "slept out." Ridding yourself of the sleep debt you've accumulated may take several days. The time you naturally start waking up tells you how much sleep you need. If you find that eight hours seems to be the average length of time you sleep on vacation, set that amount as a goal when you get home.

   Sleep experts generally agree that you need eight hours of sleep a night. People who get six or less hours of sleep have a 70 percent higher mortality rate according to the California Department of Health.

2. **Determine if you are suffering from a sleep disorder.** You want to sleep more, but sometimes it's just impossible to get a full night's rest. If excessive sleepiness is ruining your life, test yourself on the Epworth Sleepiness Scale. (Some insurance companies use this test to determine if you qualify for a referral to a sleep disorder clinic.) You can find the sleep quiz at `www.daytimesleep.org`. If you figure out that you may have a sleep disorder, you may want to get some help. You may begin by visiting your family doctor.

3. **Establish a regular sleep routine.** My dad, Jim, is a health-conscious person who always makes sure he is in bed by 10 p.m. I remember him telling me that the hours before midnight are the most important hours for rest. If you need to wake up at 6:30 a.m. and eight hours of shut-eye is your goal, you better fluff up your pillows between 10 and 10:30 p.m. Your goal should be a regular, 365-days-a-year schedule that stabilizes your internal sleep-awake biological clock.

   Sleeping longer on weekends may actually disrupt your sleep rhythms, says *Power Sleep* author Dr. James B. Maas. This disruption in your sleep routine explains why many of us suffer from the Monday-morning blahs. Sure, you "catch up" on weekends, but when Monday rolls around, your body protests when it's not allowed to sleep in.

4. **Take note of your bedroom environment.** Your bedroom needs to be dark, just the right temperature, and sleep-friendly. A double or queen-sized bed is usually too small for a couple; you may want to go for a California king-sized bed so you both have plenty of room to stretch out. (You don't want to wake up your spouse when you change your sleeping position.) If you live in a temperate climate, open a window to allow fresh air to circulate. During the winter, turn the thermostat down and throw an extra blanket on the bed. Turn your digital clock so that the red illuminated numerals don't glow directly into your eyes.

To nap or not to nap

After you have a power lunch, you feel like having a . . . power nap. Although some may say that napping is a no-no because you won't be tired at night, I find that a short afternoon nap is a wonderful way to recharge the batteries. Allow me to let you in on a professional secret: Many big-name tennis players take naps before their matches.

I once read that a 20-minute nap in the midafternoon or early evening is the equivalent of 4 hours of sleep at night. One way to power nap is to lie on the floor and place your feet on the bed or couch so that your feet are high above your body. Set an alarm for 15 to 20 minutes, close your eyes, and fall asleep. Blood travels from your elevated feet to your brain. Your feet tingle. You wake up refreshed because of the increased oxygen brought to your brain by your blood.

My husband, Mark, gives me lessons in power napping. Mark is the ultimate power napper. I see him grab a quick snooze in the back of taxi cabs, airport lounges — and planes, trains, and automobiles. Mark even schedules a regular afternoon nap into his daily planner. (He lies down on a couch in his office for a rest.) Like every change you make to be fit and healthy, you need to practice and be consistent. Napping may be one answer to your nighttime sleep problem.

5. **Be careful about exercising before bedtime.** Because physical exertion stimulates the release of adrenaline, some people cannot fall asleep after a rigorous workout. A good rule is to avoid exercising during the three-hour window *before* you plan on falling asleep. Late afternoon exercise is best if you want to ensure that you're tired, but not overstimulated; morning exercise does not seem to affect the quality of sleep. Stretching just before bedtime is fine; I sleep well after a good five-minute stretch.

6. **Watch your evening eating and drinking habits.** By now you know that coffee keeps you awake, so switch to decaf when you enjoy a dessert coffee in the evening. But the dessert may be loaded with caffeine — such as the flavoring in *gateau au chocolate doublé*. Stick to fruit-based pies and cakes after 9 p.m. if you are in the mood for sweets. And don't forget that a nightcap could be a "nightslap." Alcohol does little to improve your sleeping habits. Although a glass of wine with dinner may be fine, late-night heavy drinking may disturb your sleep. Keep in mind that heavy meals with second and third helpings just before bedtime stimulate the digestive system and keep you wound up, negatively affecting your ability to get a good night's rest.

Practice these good sleep habits and wake up raring to go. You may find that when you get enough hours of sleep, you wake up with ample energy to work out or go on a long walk *before* work — solid steps you may take to become fit.

Dealing with jet lag

Take it from someone who travels from one time zone to another many times during the year: jet lag is not a condition to be ignored. I wake up in hotel rooms at 2 a.m. — alert and ready to play a match. Unfortunately, I just went to bed three hours earlier.

I always feel the best way to deal with jet lag is to hit the ground running — right after my plane lands. I figure that a half-hour jog, a practice session on the tennis court, or a gym workout shocks my body and announces, "Listen, you're on a new time schedule here." A workout also primed my body for deep sleep that evening.

I know that some people may say that you minimize the effects of jet lag when you ease yourself into the new time zone by adjusting your sleeping and eating schedule prior to traveling. You try to parallel the new time-zone schedule for a couple of days before you depart. That approach never works for me. Whenever I get on a plane to fly across the Atlantic or Pacific, I immediately change my watch to reflect the time zone of my destination and try to adjust my eating and sleeping schedule accordingly from that point on. When I arrive, I remind myself, "Hey, you're in London. It's 9 o'clock in the morning for the Londoners, and it's 9 o'clock in the morning for me."

You may cushion jet lag by taking a mild sleep aid for the first night or two when you're on a new continent. Melatonin, Benadryl, Excedrin P.M., and others may knock you out and give you eight or nine hours of glorious sleep. After one or two nights, your body clock should be fully changed, which means you can stop using the sleep aids.

Chapter 12

Gearing Up: Exercise Clothing

• •

In This Chapter

▶ Discovering the new exercise apparel for women

▶ Outfitting the men for a workout

▶ Donning appropriate attire when exercising at home

• •

*J*ust as men and women "dress for success" in the business world, you'll feel a lot better about yourself when you wear the right workout clothes. When you look the part, you exercise with confidence, whether you're striding on a treadmill in the family den or pumping iron at the local gym. This chapter will bring you up to date on some exciting developments in fitness fashion.

Slipping into Something Comfortable: New Workout Wear for Women

Gals, you're going to like this news flash: A new style of fitness clothing is available. The style is called "lifestyle workout wear." You can wear this apparel on your way to the fitness center, while you work out, and when you shop or pick up the kids on your way home from the gym.

You may wonder how these feats may be possible. You associate exercise clothing with skintight leotards that stick to your skin when you perspire. Not any longer.

Fast-drying workout clothes? No sweat

If you last shopped for exercise clothing when Richard Simmons first began to make a name for himself, you're in for a pleasant surprise. In recent years, fitness clothing manufacturers have developed several high-tech fabrics that permit "dry wicking" — material that "wicks" away (or repels) sweat and moisture. These fabrics, produced under names such as Supplex, DryCore, and PolyDri, are being blended with small amounts of Lycra to produce the next-generation fitness wear. Not only do these scientifically designed materials wick moisture, but they also "hold" your body and don't squeeze your torso like old-fashioned spandex does.

One of the leading high-tech materials in workout wear is a Supplex/Lycra blend (86 percent Supplex/14 percent Lycra). Supplex, a cottony-soft, supple nylon fabric invented by DuPont, may be found in many cutting-edge fitness clothes for women.

In the old days, cotton shirts, polyester leotards, and cotton hose became drenched during a workout — and gave you an icky sensation when these moisture-soaked clothes clung to your skin long after you toweled off. You had to take a quick shower, lest your wet clothes made you cold and chilly. With a Supplex/Lycra blend, however, you're wearing moisture-resistant material. More good news: Just about everyone looks good in these outfits! These new workout clothes also cater to a busy mom's lifestyle. You can work out in Supplex/Lycra clothes (especially the new "bootleg" pants) and go about your overscheduled day.

I've been working out in Supplex/Lycra for some time, which means I don't interrupt my frantic day with a 30-minute shower after my workout. My workout wear of choice includes bike shorts, a tank top, and a sports bra. A simple outfit — all I need.

Investing in exercise vestments

When you're in the mood to shop for fitness clothing (and who needs a good excuse to shop?), here are some tips regarding workout wear:

- ✔ **Don't look for Supplex/Lycra at Target or Wal-Mart.** Quite frankly, Supplex/Lycra and their high-tech cousins cost more than regular fitness clothes because this clothing costs considerably more to manufacture than cotton-based clothing. This workout wear is viewed as a "specialty item" in the retail fashion world. If the store at your gym doesn't stock workout wear made with Supplex/Lycra, go onto the Internet. Type "exercise clothes," "workout wear," or "Supplex" into your search engine and surf for an online retailer. Be prepared to wade through a lot of sites.

- ✔ **Buy workout clothes that you feel comfortable wearing.** If you are dealing with "body issues" and don't want the whole world to see the shape you're in, don't wear tight bike shorts and a tank top. Ask for a "brushed" Supplex/Lycra top, which is roomier and has a softer feel. ("Smooth" Supplex/Lycra is form-fitting and hugs your body like a second skin.) You may also wear a loose-fitting, extra-large T-shirt over your fitness ensemble.

✔ **Start out with five or six articles of clothing.** You need two pairs of leggings or workout pants, which come in four lengths:

1. Bike length. These pants are short shorts.

2. Capri length. These leggings stop right below the knee.

3. Full length. These leggings reach the end of the leg.

4. Boot length. These pants are not skin tight and flare out like a regular pants leg.

✔ **You need at least two sports bras.** If you feel comfortable with your bust and stomach, you may just wear the sports bra as a top. Most women prefer to wear a long tank top over their sports bras, however. You may opt to hide your stomach by wearing a camisole over your sports bra. Some camisole tops come with built-in bras made with Lycra for extra support.

✔ **Go for solid, bright colors.** Tanks in turquoise, bright orange, lime green, and hot pink are fashionable these days. Most women wear black workout pants or leggings, but a few are working out in navy or gray versions.

✔ **View your fitness clothes as an investment.** Yes, the high-stuff costs more. You can expect to pay $35 to $75 for workout pants and leggings, $25 for bike shorts, $25 to $50 for tank tops, and $25 to $45 for bra tops. These lightweight, breathable materials don't fade, don't shrink, and keep their form. In cooler climates, you need sweatshirts, lightweight jackets, and sweatpants over your workout pants when driving to the gym or doing your errands.

✔ **Remember that you feel better when you look better.** It's fun to look sharp, and looking good may inspire you to maintain your workout routine.

Keeping the bounce to a minimum

When you reach your midlife years, the muscles in your breasts begin to lose some of their elasticity, and your breasts may appear to sag. Your breasts are made up of fatty tissue interwoven with muscle fibers called Cooper ligaments. When these resilient muscles lose their elasticity with age, I'm afraid that gravity takes over.

You may want to firm things up before hitting the exercise floor. High-impact exercises such as step aerobics or running may bounce your boobs in ways that may stretch the Cooper ligaments even further. The answer is not to batten down your chest with duct tape, but to wear a supportive "compression" sports bra (for smaller women) or an "encapsulation" bra (for well-endowed women) that keeps giggling to a minimum.

The bra seen 'round the world

I wager that half of the male population didn't know what a sports bra was until women's U.S. Soccer Team member Brandi Chastain stripped off her jersey moments after kicking in the winning goal against the Chinese in the 1999 World Cup final.

The image of Brandi exulting in her black sports bra did more than lift our spirits. She sent a message that being fit and trim is cool and that women can generate thrills on the playing field.

Perhaps Brandi's actions inspired the Berlei sports bra company to hire teen tennis diva Anna Kournikova to endorse its signature bra. When I was in England for the 2000 Wimbledon, I saw one of the 1,500 provocative billboards plastered all over Great Britain. The billboard shows Anna wearing nothing more than a sports bra and a smile with the caption: "Only the Ball Should Bounce." I'm with Anna.

Finding the right sports bra means finding a firm-support bra that totally encompasses your breasts. Your sports bra should not reveal cleavage or allow "overhang." The idea is to find a bra with cups that secure each breast and give added support. Try hopping around in front of the dressing room mirror in different styles. The "bounce" should not be painful, and your breasts should bounce a little bit even in the best sports bra. In addition, remember to check the softness of the shoulder straps and rib band and make sure no seams cross the nipple area. (These seams may cause you to develop a rash during a hard workout.)

You probably aren't aware that the fat content of your breasts increases with age: When you are in your twenties, your breasts consist of 20 to 30 percent of fat tissue. That percentage steadily grows until it reaches 90 percent in your fifties. You don't have much say in this development; the amount of fat in your breasts — as well as their size and shape — are the products of your genes.

You should replace your sports bras around every six months because their elasticity may wear out from frequent washings.

Clothes Don't Make the Man — At Least during Workouts

Okay, guys, it's your turn.

I know that "fitness fashion" is an oxymoron in the male world. I'm actually envious of males because they can work out in just about anything. I even see white-collar workers drop into clubs at lunchtime and pump a few weights —

dressed in their white-collar shirts and ties, pressed business pants, and black leather shoes.

Of course, 99.9 percent of men choose to dress up — dress down? — to work out. Men slip on old KISS T-shirts and pairs of gym shorts from their college days, and they're good to go. Fine by me. Colorwise, guys usually stick with white, black, or gray T-shirts and navy blue gym shorts.

One thing you can do, guys, is wash your T-shirts and shorts after each workout. Women would much rather smell fresh-cleaned clothes than eau de fitness. Also, stash the '70s-era "short shorts" and Speedos in a deep drawer. Believe me, you look better when your fellow exercisers don't see everything. Ditto for form-fitting bike shorts. If you could overhear women talking in the locker room, you would know that these clothing items are a turn-off, not a turn-on.

While middle-aged women worry about sagging breasts, middle-aged men must contend with some sagging of their own. Well, let me just say that you still need the same support you received the day you strapped on your first jock strap in junior high gym class. Actually, you need *more* support because muscles south of the border turn flabby with age — just as all muscles do. This change in muscle tone doesn't mean you have to wear an abdominal truss, guys. I'm just saying that you shouldn't let it all hang out when you exercise in public.

Men sometimes wonder if they should work out in boxers or briefs. Snug briefs are fine, a jock strap is even better, but boxers are a no-no because they offer zero support. Use common sense. Your privates will thank you.

Jogging Togs outside the Gym

Working out at home offers a different environment from the public gym because you may walk on your treadmill wearing nothing more than a smile and a pair of Reebok cross-trainers. (I can't say I recommend treadmilling in the buff because there is no place to hang your Walkman!)

Certainly, you don't need to impress anyone when you work out at home, but I still recommend that you dress the part. Wearing fashionable workout clothes makes a statement to yourself: I'm taking fitness seriously, and I want to look my best.

If your fitness regimen includes walking through your neighborhood, you may choose to walk in leggings or shorts. Be sure to dress in layers, especially when the temperature falls below 45 degrees. Wearing layers traps air, insulating the body from the cold. Wearing layers also enables you to adapt to the weather conditions because you may shed clothes when you become hot. Be sure to wear a jacket that you can unzip as your body warms up. Finally, wear a wool hat and mittens when the temperature is near or below freezing because you lose body heat through your head and extremities.

When you're older, you're much more susceptible to temperature changes. When the temperature is low, be sure to bundle up before you go to the gym. If you catch the flu, you may set back your fitness resolution by weeks!

Chapter 13

Finding Shoes for a Foot Over 40

● ●

In This Chapter

▶ Tracking the changes in your middle-aged feet

▶ Avoiding foot injuries

▶ Sizing up the shoe market

▶ Purchasing your athletic shoes

● ●

*J*ust as a painter needs a brush or a carpenter needs a hammer, anyone who's serious about fitness needs a pair of good shoes. The proper shoes can be the difference between comfort and discomfort, safety and injury, and getting the most out of a workout and just going through the motions.

Wearing "sensible shoes" is important to those of us over 40 because the feet change with age. Middle age is a time when the foot begins widening, the Achilles heel and ligaments on the bottom of the feet are more susceptible to tearing, and painful bunions and warts appear. The foot's arch tends to sag with the passage of years as bones soften and ligaments stretch. These developments contribute to various ailments and inflamed nerves in your foot, which is why I'm devoting a chapter to this amazing appendage. Because foot pain can cripple a fitness program faster than a four-minute mile, you should understand how to prevent foot ailments that can jeopardize your exercise regimen.

Feet Don't Fail Me Now: Problems of Middle-Aged Feet

Like cars that begin experiencing problems past the 100,000-mile mark, your middle-aged feet notice the mileage as well. Because you may have put tons of mileage on your peds by your mid-forties, I recommend that you take your feet to see a podiatrist, especially if they haven't been "running" well (groan). If you've been blessed with happy feet, you merely need to be aware of some common foot problems that crop up as you reach middle age. Let me "walk" you through them. (Sorry, I couldn't resist!)

Morton's Neuroma

When the bones of your arch sag just a tad, the nerves among the toes become compressed and inflamed. Pain — sometimes sharp, sometimes dull — is experienced each time the ball of your foot strikes the ground. This condition is called *Morton's Neuroma*.

Mike Yorkey, who's assisting me with this book, experienced Morton's Neuroma in both of his feet. After having a podiatrist specially craft inserts to raise his arches and take the pressure off his inflamed nerves, Mike continued to experience a shot of pain each time he played tennis. Mike eventually submitted to outpatient surgery in which each inflamed nerve was excised.

Other treatment methods may include administering anti-inflammatory medications such as cortisone, padding the bottom of the foot, and wearing shoe inserts.

Plantar fasciitis

If you ever experience pain on the bottom of your foot toward the heel, you may have a slight tear where the *plantar fascia* (a ligament-like band across the bottom of the foot) attaches to the heel bone, or *calcaneus*. Treatment starts with resting the foot and applying ice, followed by wearing arch supports, doing calf-stretching exercises, wearing heel cups, and taking anti-inflammatory medications.

Stress fractures

Sharp and radiating pain in the weight-bearing bones of your foot are symptoms of a fracture due to excessive stress. Resting your foot and allowing your bones to heal are common ways to treat stress fractures. Shock-absorbing arch supports and anti-inflammatory medication may help as well.

Heel bruises

Runners who constantly strike their heels on unyielding surfaces are susceptible to *heel bruises,* which are bruisings of the joints near the heel (or *calcaneus*) bones. Resting the feet and wearing new shoes or inner soles are possible remedies.

Fifty-two pickup: The bones that keep you shuffling

The human foot — with 26 bones, dozens of muscles, tendons, ligaments, and millions of nerve endings — takes the body's pounding from walking, running, or any other physical activity. Because of their weight-bearing duties, the bones of the foot are larger and stronger than those of the hand. Seven rounded bones lie below the ankle joint and form the instep, and 14 bones are in the toes (two in the big toe and three in the others). Five bones form an arch normally touching the ground only at the heel and ball of the foot.

Bunions

Bunions are bad news. A *bunion* is a bony bump, usually at the base of the big toe. Because the big toe is the hardest-working toe, every time your foot pushes off the ground, the big toe takes another hit and your bunion grows bigger and bigger. Women who wear high heels or poor-fitting shoes are at risk of developing bunions. When a bunion appears, the adjacent toes (especially the second one) can become "hammer toes" — curled or buckled upward like a claw. Hammer toes are usually not painful, but severe cases may require surgery to straighten. A surgeon's table is where many bunion sufferers eventually end up as well. A doctor shaves the first *metatarsal* (the long bone behind the big toe joint) to take away the protrusion.

Taking a Prevention Step or Two

If you don't experience any foot problems, feel free to dance a small jig. If you want to *prevent* foot problems in the future, here are some steps you can take:

- ✔ **Lose your excess weight.** The more load-bearing weight you take off your feet, the better off your feet are going to be. Foot problems may not stem from anything wrong with the feet but from carrying too much weight.

- ✔ **Women: Know that your muscles adapt to your shoes.** If you don't regularly exercise and you wear high heels to work, the muscles of your feet and legs, especially in your calves, may adapt to the shape of your high heels. When you start walking on a treadmill in cross-training shoes, your lower legs and feet muscles (especially those in your heels) readjust their lengths. You may experience pain in your calves for a couple of weeks while your muscles reshape.

✔ **Avoid overexerting yourself during some exercises.** Some exercises cause the feet to bear repeated poundings. Running and jogging are good examples of these types of foot-pounding exercises. You may be lean, but when you run, you repeatedly apply tremendous amounts of force to the feet. Try not to overdo it. I jogged *too much* during my tennis career, and now my feet are paying the price. I've suffered several serious foot injuries in recent years.

✔ **Keep your feet off concrete and asphalt.** Whether you're walking, jogging, or running, stay away from unforgiving surfaces that don't absorb some of the impact when your feet hit the ground. Cement and asphalt do not absorb shock during exercise. These hard and inflexible surfaces transmit the entire force of your feet hitting the ground to the joints of your feet, ankles, knees, hips, and lower back. Be kind to your joints and try to walk or jog in a nearby grassy park, bridal path, or golf course. Your joints will welcome a dirt or grass foundation.

For those of you fortunate to live near a beach or the sandy plain of a lakeside, walking, jogging, or running on sand is certainly a welcome respite from the concrete jungle. However, watch for the natural slope of the terrain, because a slight angulation can cause your weight to be unevenly distributed (the sides of your feet on the downhill side will absorb more pressure). This uneven weight distribution may lead to shin splints and knee pains. Keep an eye out for loose sand as well; it can cause you to turn your ankles.

✔ **Put your good walking, jogging, or running techniques to use.** When you're walking, jogging, or running correctly, pay attention to your posture by not leaning too far forward or backward. Also, make sure your entire foot hits the ground at each step.

✔ **Wear shoe inserts.** Inserts are *very* important to foot health. Using inserts is similar to aligning the wheels of a car because they provide support and cushioning, which stabilizes the feet each time they strike the pavement. Inserts come in two forms:

• **Insoles** can be purchased over the counter at drugstores. They range from inexpensive Dr. Scholl's-type pads sold in pharmacies to sophisticated versions with deep heel pockets, encapsulated air cells, and special padding. Change your shoe's insoles every three to six months. Insoles cost between $3 and $25, although sophisticated models for runners can cost more.

• **Orthotics** are custom made by a podiatrist. They are considerably more expensive than insoles; you can expect to pay between $250 and $500 to have a podiatrist outfit you with a pair. Orthotics not only provide extra support, they also subtly reshape your feet by changing your balance and the demands placed on your foot muscles. Your podiatrist may recommend orthotics to prevent your minor aches and pains from becoming serious impairments that require surgery.

If the Shoe Fits . . .

You may call them exercise footwear, tennies, athletic shoes, active wear shoes, or sneakers, but these shoes are well worth the special purchase. To slightly change a saying originally about mothers, "If the feet ain't happy, ain't nobody happy."

The sole purpose

Deciding which kind of shoes to buy is not easy these days with so many options on the market. You may purchase specialty shoes for running, walking, hiking, biking, racquetball, tennis, basketball, aerobics, weight-training, and even mountaineering.

Here's my shoe breakdown:

✔ **Tennis shoes.** Tennis shoes provide lateral stability, which means when you make quick "cutting" moves in any direction, your foot remains stable in the shoe. Good leather tennis shoes (usually $50 and up) are suitable for gym work, walking around the neighborhood, light jogging, and day hikes.

✔ **Running shoes.** Running shoes have a larger toe box and more shock absorption. Because running shoes are so light on your feet, they feel great when you walk or jog. Running shoes do not come with lateral stability, however, so any quick "cuts" may result in ankle sprains.

✔ **Basketball shoes.** A good basketball sneaker offers good traction, excellent ankle support, and firm cushioning. A basketball sneaker may be a lot of shoe for just working out in a gym (for example: walking on a treadmill) because basketball shoes weigh more than running or tennis shoes.

You throw good money away when you purchase top-of-the-line basketball shoes that run over $100. Nike, Reebok, adidas, and a host of other shoe companies target teens to purchase their obscenely priced concoctions of leather and plastic. I'm not sure why you would want to fork over big bucks for a pair of KB 8 II's (Kobe Bryant's shoe), but your kids may be clamoring for the chance.

✔ **Cross-training shoes.** Cross-training shoes are the most recent addition to the exercise shoe family. These versatile shoes fill a niche as an economical alternative to buying different shoes for every sport. Cross-training shoes work well for running, walking, racquet sports, and fitness training, including aerobics. Note: Cross-training shoes look a lot like tennis shoes.

From barely functional to highly fashionable

Shoes have come a long way, baby, in our lifetimes. Growing up, girls wore white Keds that had all the support of flip-flops. Guys strutted on the basketball court in their Converse Chuck Taylor All-Star high-tops (choice of colors: white or black) or donned baseball cleats on the ball field. Non-jocks were relegated to wearing "tennis shoes" such as Jack Purcells for outdoor play.

When the jogging boom, led by Jim Fixx (author of *The Complete Book of Running*), hit the landscape in the fall of 1977, a new market opened up for running shoes. Everyone had to have a pair of Nike or New Balance shoes with their waffle-iron soles. Then Michael Jordan and his Air Jordan Nikes came along to transform the "sneaker" industry into a billion-dollar conglomeration during the 1980s. At that time, a small British athletic shoe company noticed that growing numbers of women were attending exercise classes. These women were exercising in bare feet or in men's tennis shoes because they had nothing else to wear. Reebok responded with the Freestyle, the first athletic shoe for women's aerobic classes, and the rush was on to produce athletic shoes for different segments of the fitness world. Just as the 49ers who rushed to the California foothills 150 years ago said, "There's gold in them thar hills" — there's gold in them thar shoes.

✓ **Walking shoes.** If my book prompts you to begin a fitness regimen that starts with walking, by all means consider purchasing a pair of walking shoes. These shoes really do not differ much from tennis shoes, although some women seem to prefer their styles. Whatever turns your fashion motor on is fine with me.

I'm going to make this decision easy for you. Unless you plan on doing a lot of running (and not too many of us 40 and up do that silly stuff anymore), purchase a pair of good tennis shoes. I don't say that because I played on the Women's Tennis Association tour but because tennis shoes are the best all-around option out there. You can participate in a *lot* of different sports and physical activities wearing tennis shoes — even running. In addition, tennis shoe prices are quite reasonable because they are not viewed as specialty shoes, such as aerobics or weight-training shoes. You may find tennis shoes on sale at one of your "big box" sporting goods stores.

Shopping for shoes

New technology and a growing number of brands make buying shoes almost as difficult and confusing as buying a personal computer. The following tips guide you through this process:

✔ **Know your feet.** Your arch may have flattened out over the years, which means you need extra arch support or a larger shoe size. If your arches are high, you may need extra shock absorption in your shoes. If your ankles are weak, you may consider a basketball shoe for extra support (they are "taller" and rise up farther on your ankles).

✔ **Don't be buffaloed by the sales lingo.** Some salesperson may try to impress you with talk about "torsion boxes" and "notched-heel collars." Don't be talked into buying shoes that aren't right for you because you're too timid to admit that you don't have the foggiest idea what the salesperson is talking about.

✔ **Check your old shoes.** Look at the soles of your shoes to see where they are the most worn. If your shoes are severely worn at the outer heels or inside toe areas, ask the salesperson for shoes that are reinforced in those areas.

✔ **Buy your shoes in the afternoon**. Your feet swell during the day, so the best time to try on shoes is during the afternoon when your feet have expanded to their largest size.

✔ **Buy the proper size.** Ladies, we're famous for buying shoes one or two sizes too small just because we want our feet to look petite and narrow. The American Orthopedic Foot and Ankle Society says that 88 percent of women wear shoes too small for their feet. Wearing shoes that are too small is a surefire way to develop foot problems. Leave the tiny shoes to Cinderella.

✔ **Try on both shoes.** Maybe one of your feet has gotten slightly bigger with age, which means you might buy the wrong size if you try just one shoe on the smaller foot. Perhaps inserts can resolve any fitting problems. Consult a podiatrist for answers.

✔ **Select shoes based on your gender.** Generally speaking, women's feet are shaped slightly different than men's. Women have narrower heels, which means their heels may slip around in some men's models. You want your heels to feel anchored when you lace up the shoes.

✔ **Consider buying your shoes based on width.** New Balance is the only major athletic shoe manufacturer to produce their entire line of shoes in a full range of widths, which is one reason why podiatrists often recommend this brand. Although the core market for most sneaker companies ranges between ages 14 and 22, New Balance produces shoes with the middle-aged consumers in mind. The company keeps many past styles in production because older people tend to stick with shoe styles that they like and continue to purchase these styles for years.

✔ **Bring your insoles or orthotics to the store.** If you regularly wear inserts, you can't make a good buying decision until you try on a shoe with your inserts in place.

✔ **Try on some lightweight models.** You may find that some of the new shoes on the market are made noticeably lighter than to what you're accustomed. You may find that you prefer a lighter shoe. If you can't discern a difference between the new and old styles, you may want to purchase the less-expensive pair.

✔ **Make sure your toes can wiggle.** Bend over and press the tip of the shoes, just like you do for your young children. Wiggle your toes in the shoe's toe box while standing and sitting. You should be able to move your toes relatively freely.

✔ **Compare widths.** Note that the widest part of the shoe should correspond to the widest part of your foot. Your feet should not feel pinched as you stand or walk. The inner seams should not rub against your feet.

✔ **Make sure that your feet don't "swim" in the shoes.** Be sure to get a good fit. You need firm support when exercising. Your shoes should be roomy enough for comfort but snug enough to offer support. Walk, jump, and even jog around a bit in different shoe styles before you buy.

✔ **Check the support of the shoe.** The heel box should cradle your heel, and the shoe shouldn't buckle when you roll your ankle.

✔ **Consider Velcro snaps.** Some people prefer the convenience of Velcro snaps over conventional shoestrings for a snug fit.

You no longer have to "break in" athletic shoes. Shoes should feel comfortable on your feet before you leave the showroom floor. If your new shoes aren't comfortable in the shoe store, they're not going to be comfortable later.

Chapter 14

Getting Ready to Work Out: Warm-up Exercises

. . . .

In This Chapter

▶ A warm-up to end all warm-ups

▶ Exercises to limber up specific parts of your body

▶ Background on the International Performance Institute

. . . .

*T*o tell the truth, some fitness trainers say that stretching and warming up are the same things, while others say they are not. Some instructors advise you to warm up before you stretch, while others vouch for stretching prior to warming up. Confused? I'm not surprised. I'm here to set the record straight: Stretching and warming up are *not* the same thing.

Warming up increases the temperature and elasticity of your muscles before you start any physical activity, which includes stretching. Stretching muscles before you have warmed them up can cause tears and strains, which is why you should warm up for several minutes *before* you do any stretching movements. To do so, follow this excellent warm-up protocol designed by the trainers at the International Performance Institute. (See the sidebar in this chapter for more on the IPI.)

This comprehensive, intense warm-up regimen offers an extensive list of exercises (some of which overlap the stretching routines that I mention in Chapter 15). Be sure to carefully read the explanations and view the photos. Most "walks" or "marches" should be done for about 30 feet as I indicate. These intense exercises take about 30 to 60 minutes to complete.

Joint Mobility

A good warm-up starts with a general loosening of the neck, arms, shoulders, and trunk. Start slowly; within a few minutes, a proper warm-up should raise your body temperature by 1 to 2 degrees Fahrenheit. Warming up does more than loosen stiff muscles at your age — it can improve your ability to perform various exercises and greatly decrease your risk of injury.

✔ **Neck clock.** Rotate your head in a clockwise manner several times; then reverse direction. Move your head smoothly as it goes around and around.

✔ **Shoulder roll and shrug.** Move your shoulders in unison so that they trace a circle or oval in the air. Try this exercise with your arms down and slightly back. You should do shoulder rolls in both directions — forward and backward. After rolling your shoulders for a while, try shrugging them up and down.

✔ **Arm circle.** Extend your arms straight out from your body. Start rotating both hands at the same time, making six-inch circles. Do arm circles in both directions — forward and backward.

✔ **Arm hug.** Reach your left arm across your chest and touch the top of your right shoulder. Grab your left elbow with your right hand and push it closer to your chest, stretching the muscles in the back of your left upper arm. Reverse arms and repeat the process. (See Figure 14-1.)

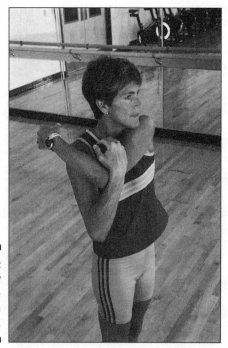

Figure 14-1: Betsy demonstrates an arm hug.

✔ **Hip crossover.** Lie on your back. With your feet off the ground and your knees bent at 90-degree angles, rock from side to side and touch your knees to the ground, keeping your knees together. (See Figure 14-2.)

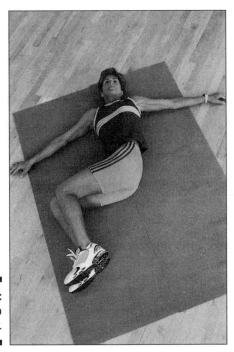

Figure 14-2:
Hip
crossover.

✔ **Leg crossover.** While lying on your back with your arms spread out, raise your right leg in the air and bring it across your body and as close to your left hand as possible. Return the leg to the starting position, and then repeat with the left leg. Continue 10 to 20 times. (See Figure 14-3.)

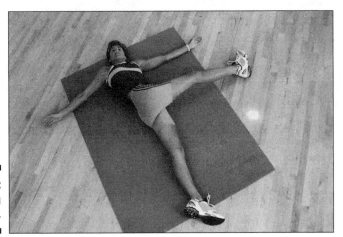

Figure 14-3:
Leg
crossover.

  ✔ **Standing trunk twist.** Rotate your shoulders as far as possible while looking behind you, allowing your arms to swing freely. Then rotate your head and shoulders to the other side of your body. (See Figure 14-4.)

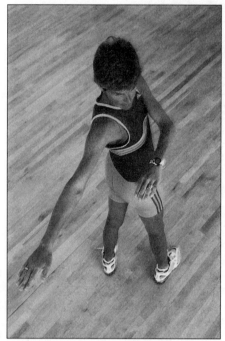

Figure 14-4:
Standing
trunk twist.

  ✔ **Standing side bend.** Interlock your fingers and place your hands on top of your head. Lean your torso to your left; then lean to your right.

Generally Speaking: Overall Warm-up Exercises

These warm-up activities — which help ready your lower body for all kinds of workouts — will increase circulation to your muscles and help you avoid muscle strains.

Ankles

These exercises ought to get your ankles good and loose:

- ✔ **Heel/toe raise.** Maintaining good posture, rock back on your heels and roll forward onto your toes. (See Figure 14-5.)

- ✔ **Heel-to-toe walk.** Place your heel on the ground; then spring up to your toes. Now switch to your other foot and repeat the action. Walk as you do these exercises for about 20 to 30 feet. (See Figure 14-6.)

- ✔ **Ankle circle.** Balance on one foot while you make circles in the air with your other foot. You can try rotating your foot below the ankle, or you can rotate the entire lower leg. You should do ankle circles in both directions, clockwise and counterclockwise.

- ✔ **Cocky walk.** Rise up on your toes; then snap the balls of the feet down while walking. Your heels should never touch the ground. Do the cocky walk for about 20 to 30 feet.

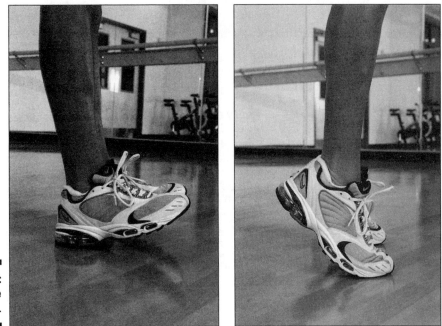

Figure 14-5:
Heel/toe
raise.

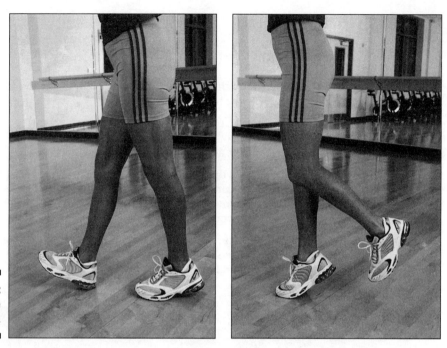

Figure 14-6:
Heel-to-toe
walk.

Hamstrings

A tight hamstring may very quickly lead to an injury that keeps you out of action for weeks and throws your whole fitness program out of whack. Take the time to warm up those "hammies." These warm-up exercises are difficult, however, so feel free to modify them according to your fitness level.

- ✔ **Hand walk.** Lean down and place your hands on the ground; then walk your hands out in front of you until your body is parallel to the ground. Keeping your legs as straight as possible, walk your hands back toward your feet. (These movements are very similar to an inchworm's movements.) (See Figure 14-7.)

- ✔ **Inverted toe touch.** Again, another difficult movement. Stand up tall as your start position. Try to raise your left leg as high as it will go and touch the toes of the left leg with your right hand. Then switch and try to raise your right foot as high as it will go, trying to touch it with your left hand. (See Figure 14-8.)

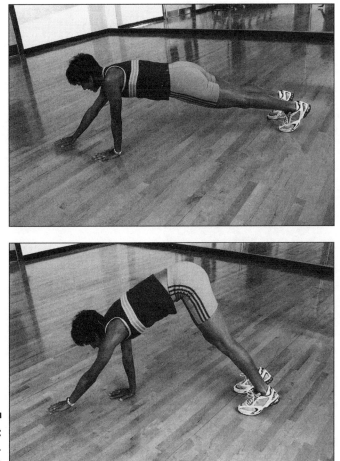

Figure 14-7:
Hand walk.

✔ **Straight leg march.** Stand up tall, keeping your chest upright. Raise your right leg straight out in front of you and try to touch your toe with your left hand and continue in a walking fashion for about 20 to 30 feet, touching your left leg with your right hand and your right leg with your left hand. These movements parallel those of a Russian dancer. Good luck with this movement. (See Figure 14-9.)

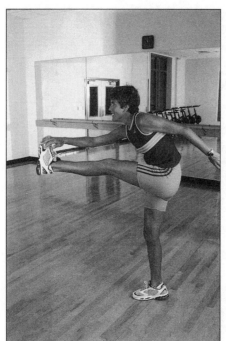

Figure 14-8:
Inverted toe
touch.

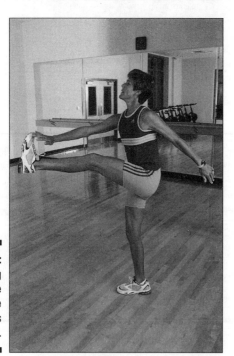

Figure 14-9:
Straight leg
march (note
that the
back is
straight).

✔ **Straight leg skip.** Same exercise as above, but add a skipping action; let your foot hit the ground twice as you move forward for about 20 to 30 feet.

Quadriceps and hip flexors

✔ **Forward lunge.** Step forward so that your front lower leg is perpendicular to the floor and your front thigh is parallel to the ground. Be sure not to let your front knee extend out over your toe; this puts undue stress on the knee. Your chest is upright and your trail leg is slightly bent. (Think of this as an exaggerated version of Groucho Marx's bounding stride.) Alternate legs while walking forward about 20 to 30 feet. (See Figure 14-10.)

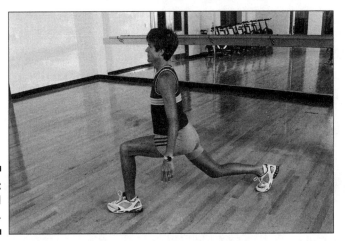

Figure 14-10:
Forward
lunge.

✔ **Backward lunge.** This movement is the same as the forward lunge, but you step backward. Although you end up placing force on the front leg, you work different muscles to get there.

✔ **Walking heel to butt.** While walking, pull your heel to your butt with your hand. Hold it for a split second until you take your next step. Try not to do this exercise with both legs simultaneously!

Hips and groin

These warm-up exercises are the keys to loosening up the middle of your frame as you prepare to work out or play the sport of your choice.

✔ **Leg cradle.** While walking, raise your right leg as if you were sitting cross-legged. Pull your right foot to the center of your body and lower it. Switch feet. Continue these movements for about 20 to 30 feet. (See Figure 14-11.)

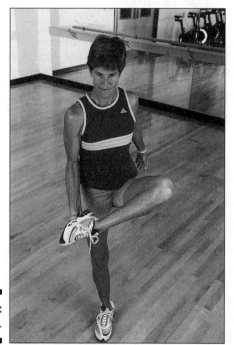

Figure 14-11:
Leg cradle.

✔ **Dog and bush.** Raise your left leg up to the side; then make a large step to the left as if you are stepping over a low fence. Repeat this with your right leg. (See Figure 14-12.)

✔ **Backward dog and bush.** This exercise requires the same movements as the dog and bush, but this time you step backward.

✔ **Lateral lunge.** Take a large step sideways to your left. Keeping your chest upright and your right leg straight, bend your left leg so that your thigh is parallel to the floor. Then stand up. Repeat three more times to the left. Then reverse back to the right. (See Figure 14-13.)

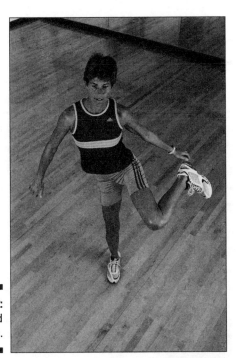

Figure 14-12:
Dog and
bush.

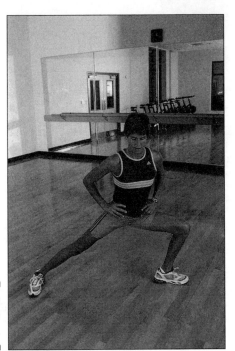

Figure 14-13:
Lateral
lunge.

Full Steam Ahead: Preparing for Forward Movement

These warm-up exercises are important because they limber up the muscles, ligaments, and tendons you use when you move forward or backward. (And don't you move forward and backward pretty frequently during the day?) You should do these movements while walking about 20 to 30 feet.

✔ **Knee hug.** Bend your leg and raise your knee to your chest; give your leg a big squeeze. Alternate this movement between your right and left legs as you walk for about 20 to 30 feet. (See Figure 14-14.)

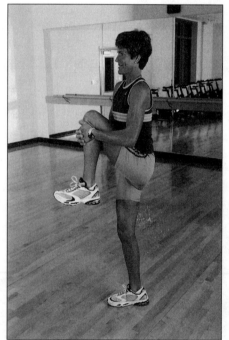

Figure 14-14:
Knee hug.

✔ **Ankle skip.** This exercise is very similar to the cocky walk, except you make a double tap with the ball of your foot.

✔ **High knee march.** Raise your knee up as high as you can and push downward and land on the ball of your foot as if you are stepping on a bug. Switch and do the same movements with your other leg. Repeat these movements as you march for about 20 to 30 feet. (See Figure 14-15.)

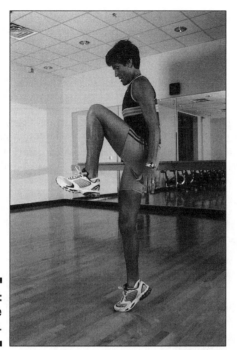

Figure 14-15:
High knee
march.

✔ **High knee skip.** Similar to the high knee march, you add a skip — a double tap on the bottom of your foot. Be sure to accentuate the downward action by thinking of stomping on a bug.

✔ **Toe up and knee up run.** This exercise requires high knee movements. Begin by standing on the toes, and then run with your knees up as high as you can, just like that old football drill. You can also do this drill without starting on your toes.

Loosening Up in Every Direction

And now for the warm-ups that get your body ready to move side-to-side and every which way but, hopefully, loose.

Lateral and base movements

✔ **Lateral high knee march.** This exercise requires the same movements as the high knee march, except you march sideways. Your main goal is to maintain a good *base*, which means keeping your feet shoulder width apart. Raise your knees up high and push with the trail leg. Repeat these movements for about 20 to 30 feet.

✔ **Lateral high knee skip.** You make the same movements as with the high knee skip, but you are skipping sideways. Be sure to accentuate the push off the trail leg. Repeat these movements for about 20 to 30 feet.

Crossovers

✔ **In-place crossover.** Mimic the Heisman Trophy position — arms out to your left side, as if you're pushing away a tackler, and left leg lifted across your body with the knee bent. Return to a base position. Perform five to ten reps. Keep your thighs close to your body. (See Figure 14-16.)

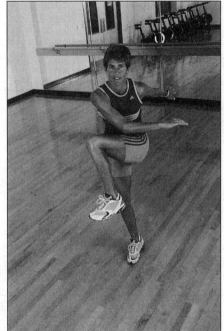

Figure 14-16:
In-place
crossover.

✔ **Carioca.** Moving sideways, cross your left leg over and step one pace to the right of your right foot. Stretch, and then return to a normal standing position. Then put your left leg behind you and cross your right foot over. Stretch, and then return to a normal standing position. Repeat the exercise several times. (See Figure 14-17.)

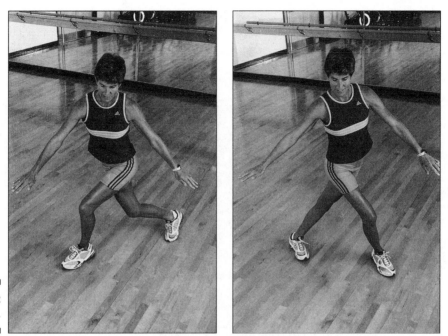

Figure 14-17:
Carioca.

Dropsteps and the backpedal

✔ **Dropstep squat.** Point your toes in opposite directions — 180 degrees. While keeping your torso upright, lower yourself so that your butt comes close to the floor, keeping your knees over your toes. Hold for one second; then stand up. Lower and raise yourself five to ten times. (See Figure 14-18.)

✔ **Dropstep bend.** With legs as nearly as far apart as possible, perform knee bends as low as you can go.

✔ **Backward reach run.** Touch your heel to your butt as you run backward.

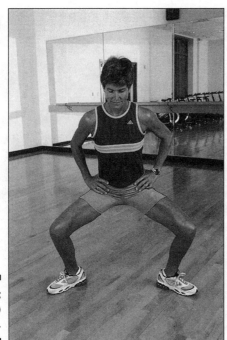

Figure 14-18:
Dropstep
squat.

What Is the IPI?

Chances are, you've never heard about the International Performance Institute, located on the grounds of the Nick Bollettieri Sports Academy in Bradenton, Florida. This "finishing school" of fitness is where world-class, tip-top athletes (Nomar Garciaparra, Kobe Bryant, and Monica Seles) go to get in even better shape.

The International Performance Institute is not just for professional athletes, however. Amateurs are welcome, and the facility sees many weekend warriors. In fact, if you ever want to get a taste —

albeit a sweaty, salty one — for what elite athletes endure on their roads to glory, the IPI trainers will be happy to work your butt off.

The IPI recommends a one-week stay. You will work out harder than you've ever worked out in your life. You will also get an education on how to stay in shape at home. For more information, contact the IPI at (941) 752-2570. You may also check out their Web site at www. zoneperformance.com.

Chapter 15

Stretching: The Overlooked Foundation of Fitness

* *

In This Chapter

▶ Following the rules to ensure safe stretching

▶ Trying a variety of stretches

▶ Discovering stretches you can do at work

▶ Avoiding outdated stretching exercises

* *

*A*fter warming up for several minutes to raise your body temperature and increase circulation in the muscles, you're ready to stretch. Stretching enhances physical fitness and reduces the risk of injury to joints, muscles, and tendons. American Flexibility Institute director Fred Dolan and I put together the following stretching program that you may incorporate into your fitness regimen. These stretches may also be your fitness workout on the days you don't have the time or inclination to walk on the treadmill or do your strength-training routine.

First, a Few Subtle Reminders

Before you get started, keep these points in mind:

> ✔ **Stretch to the point of gentle tension.** You shouldn't create pain when you stretch, but you want to stretch the muscles as far as you can *without* creating pain. Only you know how far you can stretch without causing yourself pain. You want to stretch the muscles in a slow, gradual, and controlled manner through their full range of motion. Hold your stretches for 15 to 30 seconds in the furthest comfortable position.

✔ **No bouncing!** Bouncing causes trauma to the muscles. When a muscle is damaged, it must heal itself with scar tissue. The scar tissue tightens the muscle, making you feel less flexible. When you feel less flexible, you tend to "bounce" your muscles in order to stretch. The bouncing causes more trauma to the muscles. Avoid this vicious cycle by not bouncing your muscles to begin with.

✔ **If your time is limited, hold your stretches for shorter periods of time.** The body is connected like a chain link, so if you stretch many areas for short periods, you reach your major muscle groups.

✔ **Stretch after you exercise.** I know: You spend all your energy stretching, exercising on a treadmill, and pushing some weights around. Now you're supposed to stretch *again?* Since body temperature is highest after cardiovascular exercise and strength training, stretching at this time enables you to reach your maximum range of motion.

Stretching may appear benign, but you may do some considerable damage if you're not careful. Trainers in sports clubs around the country aren't allowed to touch their clients while they stretch because of the inherent dangers in overstretching or stretching to the point of damaging muscles. Instead, trainers only instruct their clients on how to stretch. Club owners do not want to be held liable for trainers who aggressively stretch members.

Stretching Exercises

The following stretches should be done *after* warming up and *before* exercise. These stretches are easy and should be repeated several times. I include two or three versions of some stretching exercises; you may do them all or just the ones that are easier for you to do properly.

This warning bears repeating: Stretch gently without causing pain. Stretching should feel good — if it doesn't, you are stretching too far.

Calf stretch #1

Stand in an upright position; make sure your posture is good. Take a long stride with your right leg and, keeping your left heel on the floor, stretch your left calf. Control this stretch by bending or straightening your right leg. Repeat the exercise with your left leg forward in order to stretch your right calf. (See Figure 15-1.)

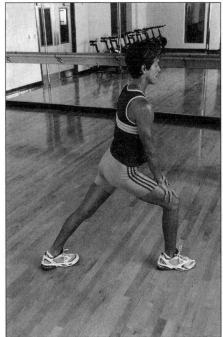

Figure 15-1:
Betsy demon-
strates calf
stretch #1.

Calf stretch #2

Stand facing a wall with your feet apart, about 18 to 24 inches from the wall. Place both of your hands on the wall and step forward with one foot, keeping your rear heel on the floor, until you can feel your calf stretch in your rear leg. Repeat this stretch with your other leg. (See Figure 15-2.)

Upper leg quadriceps stretch

Grab your right ankle and hold it with your right hand. Be sure that your hips are facing forward and that your knees are next to each other. (You may find that keeping your balance is difficult; if so, use a wall or chair for support.) Repeat this stretch by grabbing your left ankle with your left hand. Be sure not to twist your shoulders. (See Figure 15-3.)

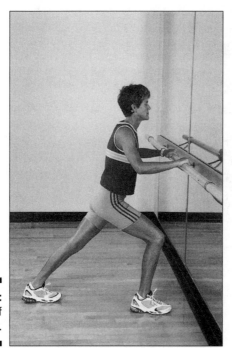

Figure 15-2:
Calf
stretch #2.

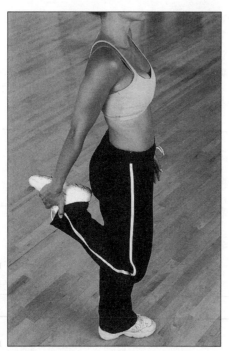

Figure 15-3:
Upper leg
quadriceps
stretch.

Inner thigh stretch

Stand with your feet apart and hands on your upper thighs. Straighten your left leg and bend your right leg to stretch your inner thigh. Your feet should point straight ahead. Now switch and stretch the other inner thigh. Keep your upper body fairly still. You may switch from side to side after holding the stretch for several seconds on each side. (See Figure 15-4.)

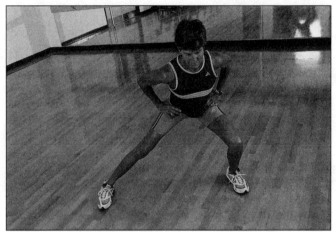

Figure 15-4:
Inner thigh
stretch.

Leg stretch #1

Sit on the floor and, holding your ankles, pull the soles of your feet together. Keeping your back straight and erect, gently pull your heels toward your groin and press your knees toward the floor. You can feel your groin stretch. (See Figure 15-5.)

Leg stretch #2

Sit on the floor and pull your right heel into your groin area while extending your left leg. Lean over your extended leg and reach out as far as you can. Feel the hamstrings and lower back stretch. If you can reach your ankle, you're highly flexible. Advanced stretchers can point their feet as they reach, which stretches more muscles. Be sure to repeat the stretch on the other side of your body. (See Figure 15-6.)

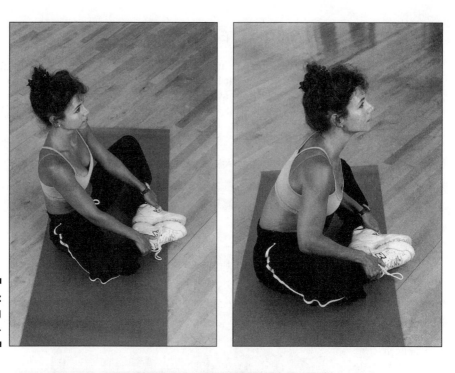

Figure 15-5:
Leg
stretch #1.

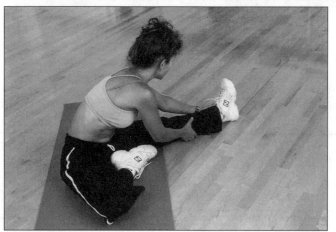

Figure 15-6:
Leg
stretch #2.

Leg stretch #3

While standing, take a large step forward into a lunge position. Make sure your front knee remains over your foot and ankle and does not extend out past your toes. Lower your back knee toward the floor, keeping your torso upright. Feel your front hip area stretch. Repeat the exercise with the other leg forward. (See Figure 15-7.)

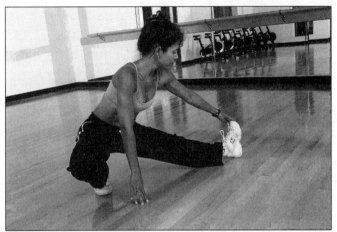

Figure 15-7: Leg stretch #3.

Leg lift #1

Kneel on the ground and relax. Place your hands on the floor in front of you, keeping your weight evenly distributed. Lift your right knee to the side until your right leg — from your knee to your hip — is roughly parallel to the ground. Make sure your right hip doesn't rise up when you lift your right knee; your right knee and right hip should be aligned fairly horizontally. Repeat the exercise with your left leg. (See Figure 15-8.)

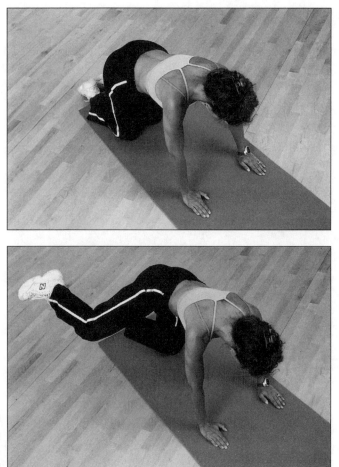

Figure 15-8:
Leg lift #1.

Leg lift #2

Lie on your side in a relaxed position with your knees slightly bent. Put one arm under your head. Raise your upper leg while keeping your knees slightly bent. Now perform this exercise on the other side of your body. (See Figure 15-9.)

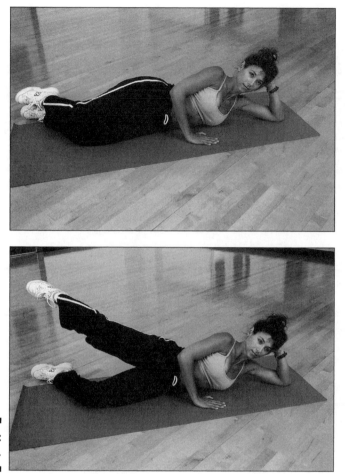

Figure 15-9:
Leg lift #2.

Leg lift #3

While continuing to lie on your side, straighten your upper leg and lift it as far as you comfortably can. Don't be discouraged if you can't lift your leg too far. Repeat this stretch with your other leg. (See Figure 15-10.)

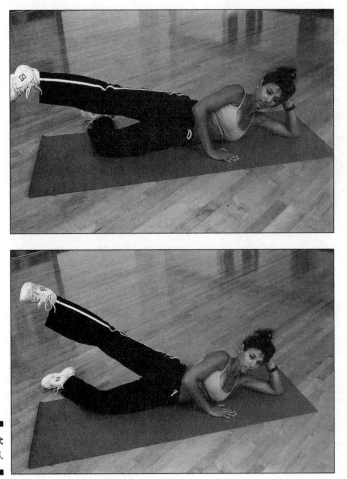

Figure 15-10:
Leg lift #3.

Lower back stretch

Lie on your back with your legs straight. Bend your right leg and pull your knee toward your chest with your hands holding the back side of the leg. Repeat this stretch with your other leg. (See Figure 15-11.)

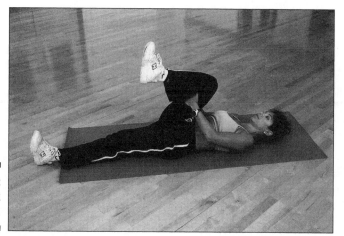

Figure 15-11:
Lower back
stretch.

Adding Some Life to Your Workday

Today's workplace environment — Cubicle City with 8'x 8' partitions — is not fitness friendly. You sit for hours at a time, hunched before your computer monitor, not moving at all, except for your right hand operating the mouse.

You need stretch breaks! Even the most slave-driving boss shouldn't mind your standing up and limbering your muscles. A stretch break increases your productivity, elevates your blood flow, warms your muscles, and helps you feel better while you do your job.

The following stretches — which can be done in business attire — may be done in your cubicle, employee break room, or corporate fitness center. Hold each stretch for ten to 20 seconds. Repeat three or more times. Do these stretches at least once every two hours (although once an hour is optimal.)

These stretches also work well on plane trips On your next cross-country excursion, get up and stretch at 39,000 feet. You need to stretch with the way seats are jammed up next to each other in coach. You may stretch in the rear of the plane (where the lavatories are). Don't let your muscles tighten up in your cramped seat 42B!

Stretches for the shoulders and neck

- ✔ With hands on your hips, move your head slowly from side to side. Avoid rolling your head. Feel the stretch in your neck muscles.

- ✔ Move your head slowly from back to front. Feel the stretch in your neck muscles. Remember to keep the movements gentle; don't allow your head to drop all the way back.

Stretches for the shoulders, chest, and upper back

- ✔ Reach your right arm straight up toward the ceiling; let your other arm remain at your side. You should feel this stretch all the way down your right arm and the right side of your body. Repeat the stretch by switching your arms.

- ✔ Hold your arms straight in front of you and make small circles from the shoulder. Then make reverse circles. You should feel the stretch in both arms.

- ✔ While standing, place your right palm and forearm against the wall. Rotate your torso away from that arm until you feel a stretch across your chest and shoulder. Repeat this with the left arm.

Stretches for the thighs and hips

- ✔ Stand on your right leg and lift your left foot behind you with your knee bent. Pull your left foot up gently with your left hand. Be sure your right knee is not locked; keep it slightly bent. Repeat this stretch with your left leg. You may steady yourself by holding on to a chair or leaning against a wall with your free hand. (This is similar to the upper leg stretch, described earlier in this chapter.)

Stretches for the calves and ankles

- ✔ Stand facing a wall (about 18 to 24 inches from the wall) with your feet apart. Place one foot slightly in front of the other. Put both hands flat against the wall and lean toward it until you feel the calf stretch in your rear leg. Repeat this stretch with your other leg. (This is basically the same exercise as calf stretch #2, described earlier in this chapter.)

Flex appeal

A few years ago, American Flexibility Institute director Fred Dolan asked me to try a stretching apparatus that he developed called the StretchMate. I liked it so much that the StretchMate now occupies a corner of my bedroom. This equipment serves as a visible reminder that I need to stretch. I consistently stretch for at least five minutes just before I go to bed.

The StretchMate looks like some 21st century spider web (see photo), but it's surprisingly effective and helps me stretch to levels that I never reached before. This weblike device of steel tubing and rubber cords enables you to stretch in any position. The Boston Celtics have one in their training room, and a StretchMate travels with the Ladies Professional Golf Association (LPGA) Tour. Dance troupes like Baryshnikov Productions and the American Ballet Theatre swear by them.

Fred predicts that you'll see more and more StretchMates in fitness clubs around the country. Call (508) 429-0707 for more information or write: StretchMate, 24 Water St., Holliston, MA 01746

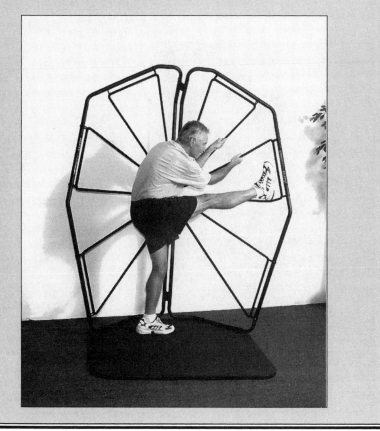

Stretches for the lower back and lower leg

✔ Stand with your feet apart and one leg ahead of the other. Place your hands on your hips. Your rear knee should be slightly bent. Straighten your rear knee until you feel the stretch in the calf and lower leg muscles. Repeat with your other leg forward. (See Figure 15-12.)

✔ The following exercises must be done on the floor or ground, which may be impossible in certain types of work clothes:

  • Lie on your back with your knees straight. Lift your right leg with your knee bent and pull it toward your chest. Repeat this with your left leg. (This is similar to the lower back stretch, described earlier in this chapter.)

  • Sit on the floor with your right leg curled in front of you and your left leg extended in front of you with the knee bent. Gently lean forward. Feel the stretch in your left hamstring and lower back area. Repeat this stretch with your other leg. (See Figure 15-13.)

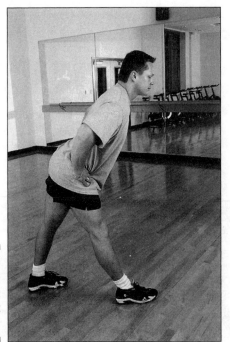

Figure 15-12:
A lower leg stretch you can do at work.

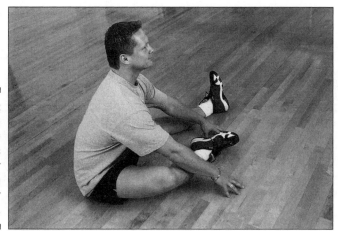

Figure 15-13:
This simple exercise stretches your hamstring and lower back.

The Seven Deadly Stretches

Some of the stretches you learned in grade school or aerobic classes are now *verboten*, says Fred Dolan. You should deep-six any of the following stretching exercises. (I couldn't even bring myself to ask a model to demonstrate them, so Fred supplied some drawings of these dangerous maneuvers.)

1. **The yoga plough.** Whoever thought that letting the neck support the weight of the body was crazy. This movement may damage the vertebrae, stretch ligaments dangerously, and even injure your spinal cord. (If there is one thing you want to avoid in life, that would be injuring your spinal cord.) An older person may even induce a stroke because this movement on the spinal cord may cut off blood to the brain. (See Figure 15-14.)

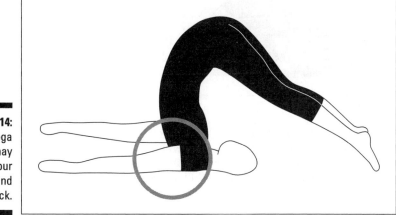

Figure 15-14:
The yoga plough may harm your back and neck.

2. **The knee stretch** (also called sitting on your haunches). This stretch may damage the ligaments on both sides of your knee. Ligaments support your joints and, once stretched, these ligaments do not spring back. Over time, this stretch may result in chronic knee problems. (See Figure 15-15.)

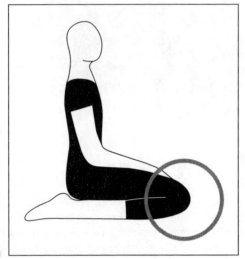

Figure 15-15:
This knee stretch is a good way to damage your knee ligaments.

3. **The sit-and-reach stretch.** This popular stretch may cause lower-back strain, especially for those who "bounce" during this movement. You may initially feel good stretching your back this way, but you don't feel good when you damage your lower back. (See Figure 15-16.)

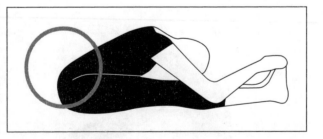

Figure 15-16:
The sit-and-reach stretch: popular, but potentially dangerous.

4. **The toe touch.** Remember this exercise from the elementary school play yard? This bomb-shelter–era stretch appears benign, but when you bend at your waist, your abdominal muscles don't work, and the vertebrae in the lumbar area are rendered unstable. You're a candidate for chronic lower-back pain with this stretch. (See Figure 15-17.)

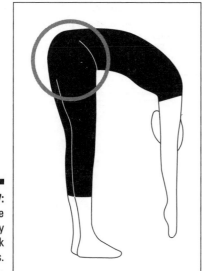

Figure 15-17:
This toe
touch may
lead to back
problems.

5. **The stiff leg raise.** If you do a double leg raise and your back arches, that result means your abdominal muscles are not strong enough for this exercise. The arch indicates that your back is being pulled by the *psoas major* (hip flexor muscles) or a combination of muscles, which strains the lower-back muscles. (See Figure 15-18.)

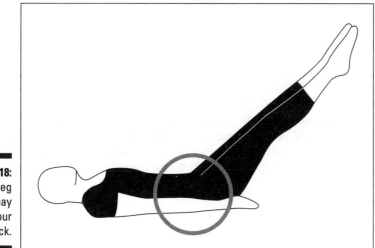

Figure 15-18:
The stiff leg
raise may
strain your
lower back.

6. **The wide-stance alternating toe touch.** This staple from junior high P.E. is not only bad for your back, it can cause a groin injury because the wide stance strains the ligaments in your lower back. (See Figure 15-19.)

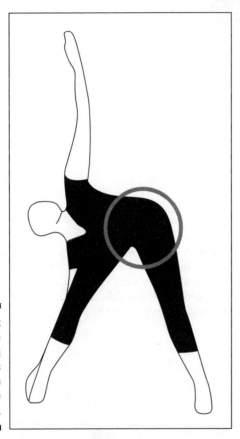

Figure 15-19: These alternating toe touches are a groin injury in the making.

7. **The single- or double-inverted hurdler's stretch.** If you are a runner, you probably do some variation of the hurdler's stretch. Forget this version, which twists and compresses the kneecap and improperly stretches the medial ligaments of the knee. (See Figure 15-20.)

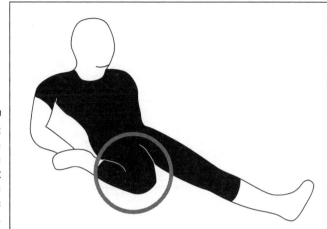

Figure 15-20:
Knee
damage
may result
from these
hurdler's
stretches.

Chapter 16

Working Your Upper Body

*A*fter you stretch like Gumby and warm up like sprinter Marion Jones, you may be ready for a rest.

That's fine! But as you consider *how* you're going to become fitter and shed excess weight, sooner or later you find that you need to do some strength training. Strength training is important, especially if you want to travel through the second half of your life with a minimum of discomforts and risks of injury. (I talk more about the need for strength training in Chapter 6.)

Strength-Training Basics

As you start your exercises to improve your tone and strength, keep in mind these pointers:

✔ **Don't lift or push too fast.** You should do your repetitions in slow to moderate speeds. Repeating the movements at a slow to moderate speed helps you to fully contract your muscles through their full range of motion. If moving slower means you lift fewer plates, so be it. You need discipline to move slowly and maintain proper form. Those guys you see grunting and groaning while they "throw" heavy weights are at a greater risk of hurting themselves because they employ poor form. Throwing weights and moving fast introduces momentum into movements, which makes the exercises less productive and less effective.

✔ **Go for eight to 12 repetitions before stopping.** Be sure you are not lifting too many plates; you should be able to do at least eight reps. If you're just beginning, make it just one set. (One set of reps may be all you need; see Chapter 6). If you're going to complete two sets, be sure to rest for one or two minutes between sets.

✔ **Take longer *finishing* the repetition.** Some people take their time lifting up, and go way too fast on the down motion. A reasonable pace is one or two seconds for the lifting portion of the exercise, and three or four seconds for the lowering portion of the move. Fast, jerky movements substantially increase the likelihood of an injury.

✔ **Lift to the point of fatigue.** Many people think that strength training is lifting to the point of failure. Wrong! You want to lift the point of fatigue. When you're over 40, the chances of injuring yourself are much greater when you lift to the point of failure.

✔ **Remember to breathe out while lifting weights.** Holding your breath and clenching your teeth tightens muscles and increases blood pressure. Exhale when your muscles contract or at the time of exertion.

✔ **Work your larger muscle groups first — chest, back, and legs.** Then move into the smaller muscle groups — shoulders, arms, and calves.

✔ **Do your strength training in 60 minutes or less.** Unless you harbor aspirations of becoming the next Mr. Universe, senior division, you should finish doing the circuit in less than an hour.

✔ **Lift at least twice a week, but not two days in a row.** Once you hit middle age, your fatigued muscles need about 48 hours to rebuild.

✔ **Save your abdominal work for last.** The body is good and warm by then. You don't want to tear an abdominal muscle.

Dumbbell Exercises For Dummies

Even with dumbbells, you want to train muscle groups from large to small, with the abdominal muscles last. Find a pair of dumbbells that are a comfortable weight for you — probably 2.5 or 5 pounds — and try these exercises, in order:

1. **Shoulder shrug.** With weights in your hands and your hands at your sides, shrug your shoulders. Do a set of eight to 12 repetitions.

2. **Arm raise.** Hold weights in your hands and your hands at your sides; then extend one arm to shoulder height. Hold for a couple of seconds before extending the other arm. (See Figure 16-1.)

3. **Arm swing.** Tennis players and golfers appreciate this drill. Swing one arm in a pendulum motion, mimicking the swing of a golf club or tennis racket. (See Figure 16-2.)

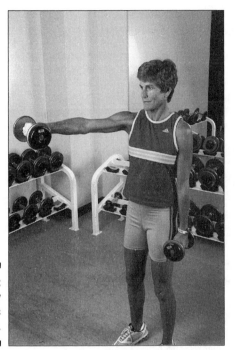

Figure 16-1:
Betsy
demonstrates
the arm raise.

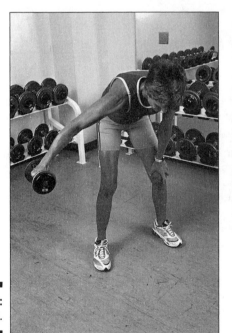
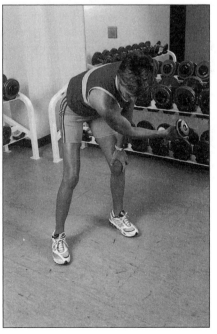

Figure 16-2:
Arm swing.

4. **Arm curl.** Let your arms hang at your side while you clutch the dumbbells. Lift both hands in front of you toward your shoulders with your
   elbows bent. Do a set of eight to 12 repetitions. (See Figure 16-3.)

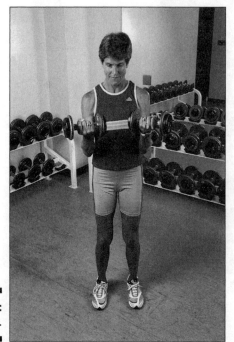

Figure 16-3:
Arm curl.

5. **Arm behind the neck.** (You may want lighter dumbbells for this exercise.) Holding a light weight, place your hand behind your head. Lift the
   weight straight up and down until your arm is tired. Repeat the motion
   with your other arm holding a light weight. (See Figure 16-4.)

6. **Arm drop.** Let your arms hang at your side while you clutch the dumbbells. Let one arm drop alongside your thigh as you bend over to the
   side. Straighten up and repeat the motion on the other side of your
   body. Do a set of eight to 12 repetitions. (See Figure 16-5.)

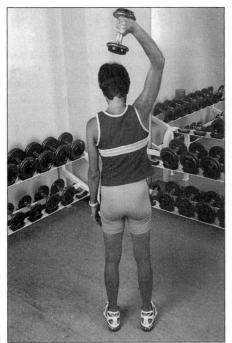

Figure 16-4:
Arm behind
the neck.

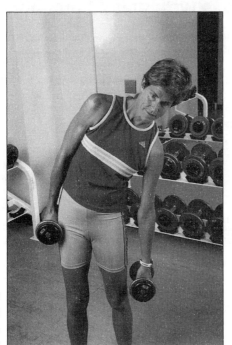

Figure 16-5:
Arm drop.

Working the Weight Machines

Listen up, everybody: Strength machines are to fitness what the computer is to word processing. Weight machines like the Nautilus, Hoist, Cybex, and Pace produce three times the results in *one-tenth* of the time. (Chapter 7 contains descriptions of these machines.)

Using these strength machines is as easy as counting 1-2-3. When working my upper body, I'm partial to the following strength-training exercises and machines.

- **Chest press.** This staple for upper-body development is good for developing your chest muscles, as well as your shoulders and triceps. (See Figure 16-6.)

- **Incline chest press.** This exercise works the upper half of your chest and anterior shoulder. (See Figure 16-7.)

- **Pec fly.** This exercise employs an excellent fundamental movement that develops overall chest strength. Make sure to keep the back of your head on the bench. (See Figure 16-8.)

FAST FACT

A name synonymous with weight machines

We can thank Arthur Jones for revolutionizing weight training. After 20 years of experimentation, in 1970 he developed the first strength machine — a pullover machine for muscles in the torso — that provided *variable resistance.* Using carefully designed spiral pulleys or "eccentric cams," the machine compensated for changes in leverage throughout a joint's range of motion and applied more consistent resistance throughout the exercise, allowing more muscle fibers to be involved.

Arthur looked at those cams and said to himself, "You know what? That looks like a nautilus shell." And a company name was born. In slightly more than 30 years, Nautilus has almost become a generic word (much like Kleenex or Xerox) for the strength-training machines you see on the floors of health clubs from Portland, Maine, to Portland, Oregon.

These days, Nautilus is showing some gray in its whiskers, and upstarts such as Hoist, Cybex, and Pace are nipping at its heels. I've worked out on several different brands, and it's hard to pick one over another. I can tell you, though, that these amazing machines are the cornerstone of anaerobic fitness.

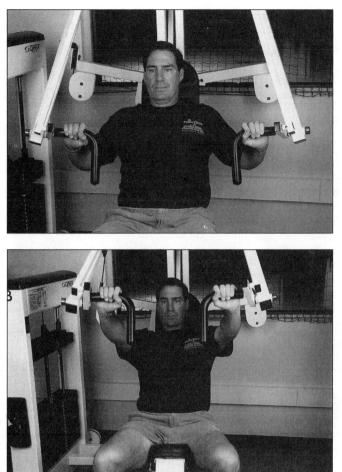

Figure 16-6:
Chest press.

✔ **Seated row.** This exercise works the major muscle groups of the back —
the *latissimus dorsi* (one of the two broad, flat, triangular muscles running from your vertebral column to your upper arm) and the lower
trapezius (back muscles that allow you to raise your head and shoulders). Don't overstretch; finish this movement with your spine erect.
(See Figure 16-9.)

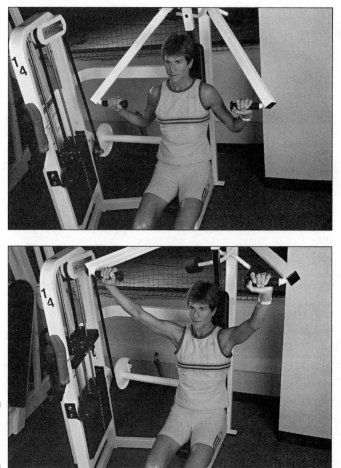

Figure 16-7:
Incline
chest press.

✔ **Lat pulldown.** Same movement as in the seated row, but from a different angle. Lean back slightly, keeping your chest up and your shoulder back as you pull the bar to your chest. This exercise is a good one to help develop that V-shaped, tapered look and strengthen your muscles that keep your body from slouching forward. (See Figure 16-10.)

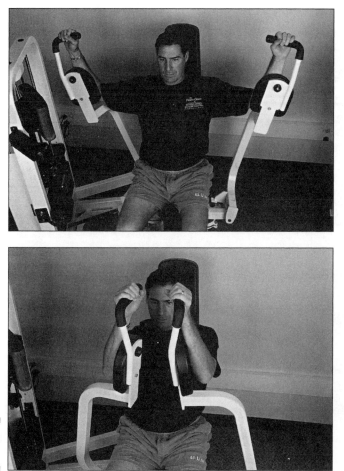

Figure 16-8:
Pec fly.

✓ **Shoulder press.** This exercise works the shoulders and upper-back muscles. You may protect your lower back from compression by contracting
your abdominal muscles. (See Figure 16-11.)

✓ **Lateral raise.** Tired of wearing shoulder pads? Then you'll love this
machine. When lifting from your elbows, you work your deltoid muscles.
Working your deltoid muscles is ideal for developing your shoulders.
This exercise also helps you achieve that V-shaped, tapered look. Be
sure to relax your shoulders while you lift your elbows toward the ceiling. (See Figure 16-12.)

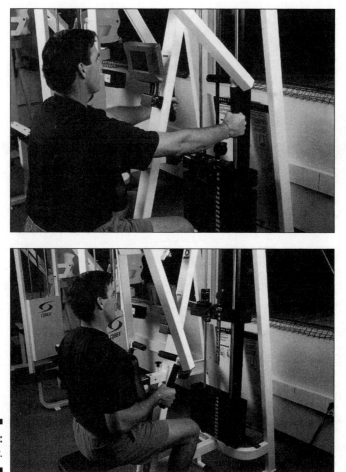

Figure 16-9:
Seated row.

✔ **Tricep extension.** This exercise develops the triceps and is a great flab fighter for the back of the arms! Be sure to keep the upper arms still and close to your sides while performing this exercise. (See Figure 16-13.)

✔ **Preacher curl.** Rounding out your upper-arm workout is this exercise that isolates the biceps and is a must for developing upper-body strength. Make sure you alternate your movements, working both of your arms. (See Figure 16-14.)

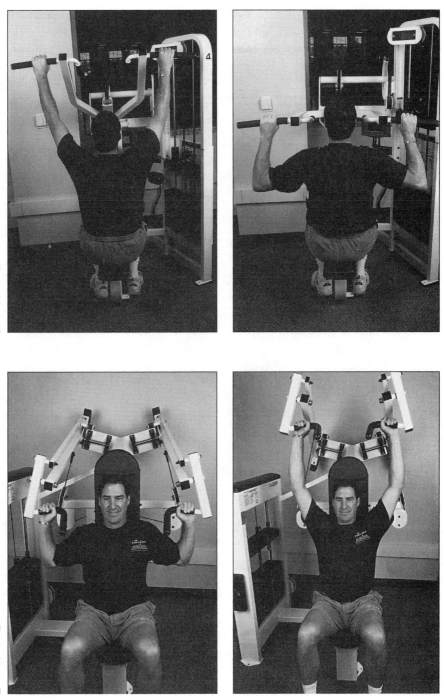

Figure 16-10:
Lat
pulldown.

Figure 16-11:
Shoulder
press.

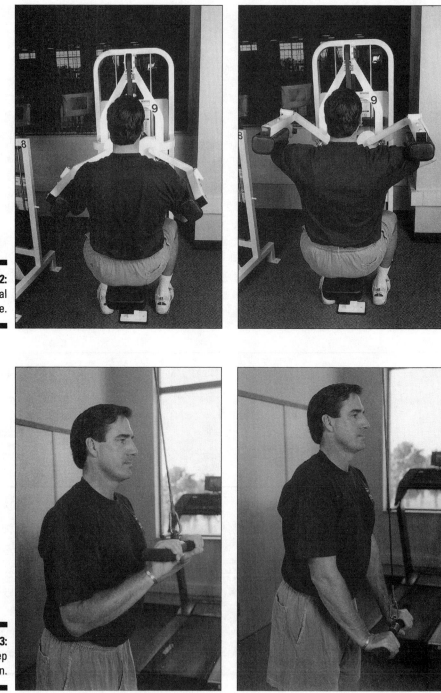

Figure 16-12:
Lateral raise.

Figure 16-13:
Tricep extension.

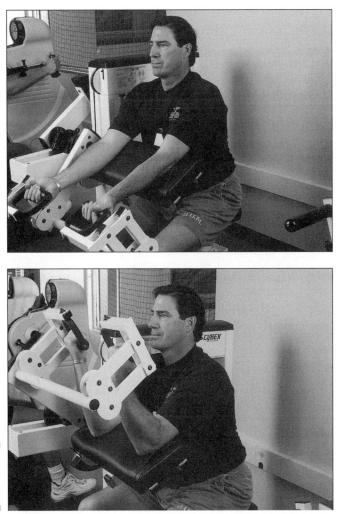

Figure 16-14:
Preacher
curl.

Chapter 17

Working Your Legs and Lower Torso

*M*any people equate strength training with working the arms, shoulders, and chest, so overlooking the lower torso — trunk, abdominal muscles, lower back, thighs, and legs — is easy to do.

The makers of weight equipment haven't overlooked the lower body, however, and neither should you. This chapter focuses on the exercises that strengthen the stomach and lower back; strong muscles in both areas can help you deal with that modern-day scourge, a sore back.

(I'm not including instructions on how to use cardiovascular equipment that works the lower extremities — treadmills, steppers, and stationary bikes — in this chapter because you already know how to walk, climb stairs, or pedal a bike. But if you're not sure how to use a certain aerobic machine, a fitness trainer or health club employee will gladly give you a demonstration.)

Before you start these exercises, be sure to review the strength-training pointers in Chapter 16. Now, let's get right into strength training for the lower body.

Hitting below the Belt

These exercises hold the key to developing tone and strength in your legs and hips:

✔ **Inverted leg press.** Believe it or not, this exercise is safer than a squat with free weights and gives overall development to the body. Start with lighter weights to give the legs a nice pump before you move on to other exercises. The inverted leg press is a good finishing exercise as well. (See Figure 17-1.)

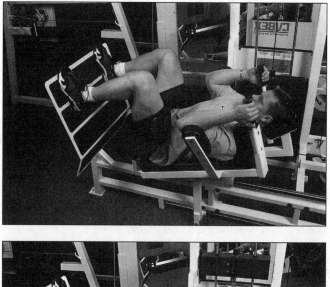

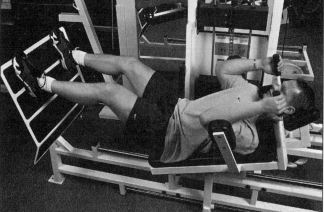

Figure 17-1: Inverted leg press.

✔ **Leg extension.** Leg extensions develop the quadriceps for lower-body power and are perfect for defining the front of the thigh. Be sure to keep your back against the pad and toes pointing up, extending the knees fully. (See Figure 17-2.)

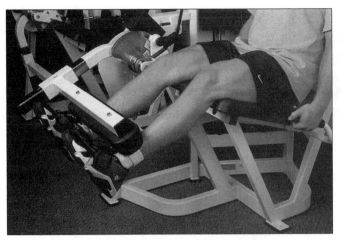

Figure 17-2:
Leg
extension.

✔ **Lying leg curl.** This exercise uses the hamstrings, a sensitive muscle group, so keep the weight on the lighter side. Lie on your stomach with your kneecaps just off the bench. Exhale as you press your hips down and curl your heels up to your buttocks. Lower your legs slowly, keeping the weight under control. Use a full range of motion and breathe. Don't neglect this exercise, because you need to keep balance with its opposing muscle group, the quadriceps. (See Figure 17-3.)

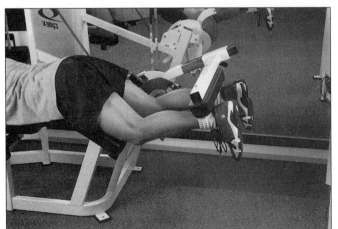

Figure 17-3:
Lying
leg curl.

✔ **Seated leg curl.** This is the same exercise as the lying leg curl, only in an upright seated position. Keep your hips in a neutral position and your back against the pad as you flex your knees, bringing your heels as close to your buttocks as possible. (See Figure 17-4.)

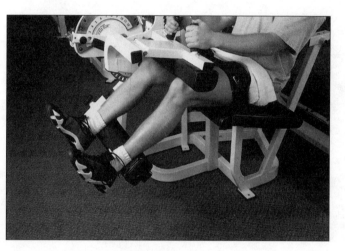

Figure 17-4:
Seated
leg curl.

✔ **Seated calf press.** This exercise works another sensitive muscle that should not be overworked or overlooked: the calf muscle. Let the weight give you a good stretch, then rise up on the balls of your feet as far as possible before slowly lowering yourself. (See Figure 17-5.)

✔ **Hip adduction.** This exercise works the inner thigh as you squeeze your knees together. Use lighter weights with this exercise. Go slow and do a higher number of reps. (See Figure 17-6.)

Hearing pops and crackles is common, so don't be alarmed; the pubic bone sometimes needs to adjust as connective tissue separates.

✔ **Hip abduction.** In this exercise, you will push your knees out and away from each other. You'll feel this exercise the next day, but working the outer hip muscles is important. Doing hip abductions stabilizes the pelvic muscles. (See Figure 17-7.)

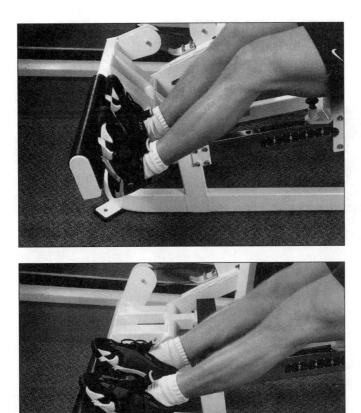

Figure 17-5:
Seated
calf press.

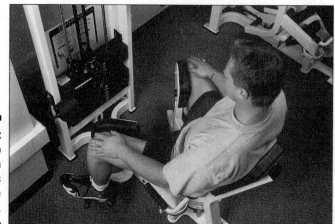

Figure 17-6:
Hip
adduction
(note pads
on inside
of knees).

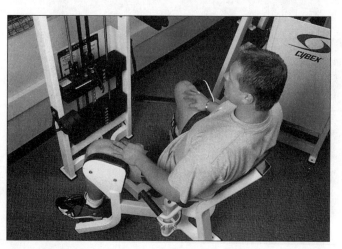

Figure 17-7:
Hip
abduction
(note pads
on outside
of knees).

✔ **Super lunge.** Let's hop off the strength-training equipment now. You know how you feel regular lunges the next day? Wait until you make lunges with dumbbells in your hands! When making a lunge, step forward so that your front lower leg is perpendicular to the floor and your front thigh is parallel to the ground. Don't put extra stress on your front knee by letting it extend out over your toes. Good technique also means keeping your chest upright and your trailing leg slightly bent. (See Figure 17-8).

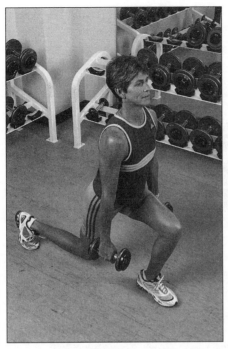

Figure 17-8:
Betsy
performs a
super lunge.

Tuning Up the Torso

These low-tech exercises may not use a strength machine, but they'll help keep your abdominal muscles (abs) and back in good condition:

- ✔ **Low ab tilt.** This basic exercise focuses on developing the lower abdominal muscles, reducing the paunch, and supporting the lower back. Keep your back as flat as possible as you bring your knees to your chest. Repeat this five to ten times. (See Figure 17-9.)

- ✔ **Ab crunch.** Six-pack attack! This basic exercise develops the upper abdominal muscles. Don't use your hands to pull your head and neck up; just reach for your knees. Keep your feet flat on the floor. (See Figure 17-10.)

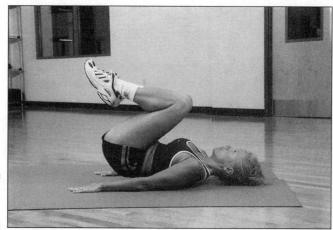

Figure 17-9:
Low ab tilt.

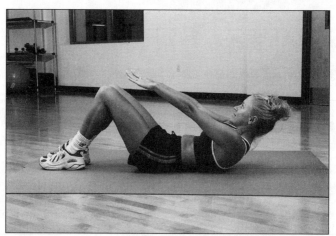

Figure 17-10:
Ab crunch.

✔ **Prone back extensions.** Lying face-down on the floor, lift your chin to bring the back of your head to your upper shoulders. Press your hands into the floor. Contract your upper spinal muscles and lift your torso until your belly button is just off the floor. Be sure to contract your gluteal muscles to protect your lower back. Don't lock your elbows! (See Figure 17-11.)

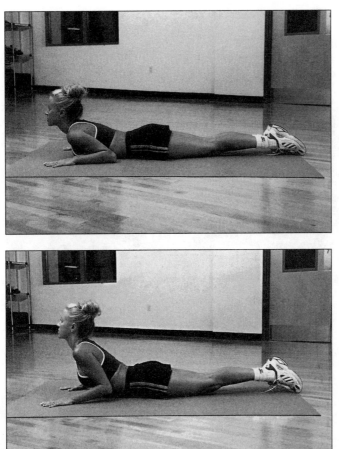

Figure 17-11:
Prone back
extensions.

Getting on the Ball

You may enjoy using a giant, soft rubber exercise ball — such as the Gymnic Swiss Ball — for strength exercises, improving balance and coordination, and increasing flexibility. You may see one or two of them at health clubs. While exercise balls are a fun way to break up an exercise routine, you won't build an entire workout around one.

Jumbo exercise balls, which come in bright, fluorescent colors and various sizes, were originally used by Swiss therapists to treat children with cerebral palsy by enhancing their balance and strength. Everyone can benefit from this new fitness craze. You try to stay upright on the ball while maintaining good posture and alignment. That's not easy to do, as I can attest. Just try doing push-ups with your legs resting on the ball!

Here are some exercises you can try on the ball:

✔ **Ab crunch on the ball.** Here's a creative exercise for the upper abdominals that allows for a greater range of motion than doing a crunch on the floor. (See Figure 17-12.)

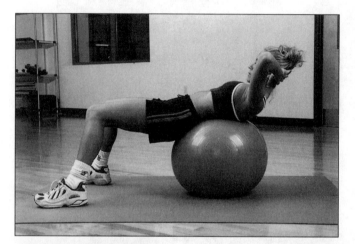

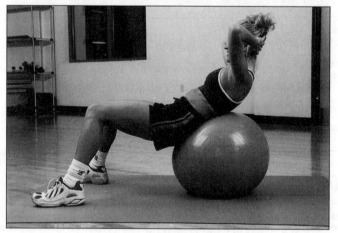

Figure 17-12:
Ab crunch
on the ball.

✔ **Lower back extension on the ball.** This exercise is a safe and effective way to strengthen the musculature of the lower and upper back from hip to shoulder. (See Figure 17-13.)

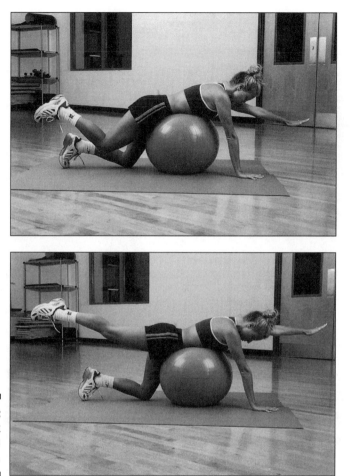

Figure 17-13:
Lower back
extension
on the ball.

✔ **Hamstring stretch on the ball.** You can't beat this exercise — it's easier
than sitting on the floor, and you get a great stretch for the back of the
leg. (See Figure 17-14.)

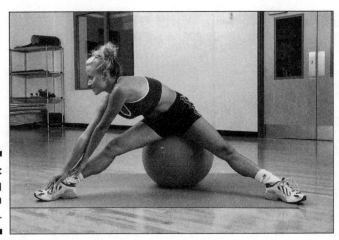

Figure 17-14:
Hamstring
stretch on
the ball.

✓ **Pose of the child.** Try this exercise to stretch the back and calm the mind (because it's so relaxing). This is a good one to do after the prone back extensions. (See Figure 17-15.)

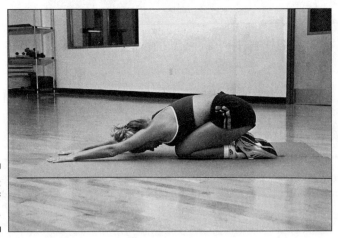

Figure 17-15:
Pose of
the child.

Chapter 18

Oh, the Pain: Avoiding Injuries

● ●

In This Chapter

▶ Understanding "boomeritis"

▶ Understanding your aging muscles

▶ Avoiding injuring yourself

▶ Knowing heart attack symptoms

● ●

*I*njuries can happen to anyone. Even world-class athletes can fatigue, strain, sprain, or — heaven forbid — tear a muscle, tendon, or ligament. (I know I've had my share of injuries over the years, including a tournament-ending foot problem at the 2000 Wimbledon when I was playing in an "old ladies" doubles event.) But these types of injuries are certainly more *likely* to happen to those of us in our forties, fifties, and sixties.

In this chapter, I show you how common injuries are in middle-aged exercisers, explain why we are more susceptible to injuries in our advancing years, and offer some tips to help you stay out of the doctor's office. I also give you the warning signs of the most serious "injury" of all — a heart attack.

Injuries — More Common Than the Cold

According to the U.S. Consumer Product Safety Commission (CPSC), sports-related injuries to baby boomers increased 33 percent during the 1990s, which had a considerable impact on health-care costs for the nation.

Unfortunately, injuries are so common for today's forty-somethings and fifty-somethings that we have a special name for it: *boomeritis.* Dr. Nicholas A. DiNubile, a Philadelphia orthopedic surgeon and sports medicine expert, is credited with inventing the term. He coined boomeritis after noticing all the "itises" he was seeing in middle-aged patients — tendonitis, bursitis, arthritis, and so on. He also observed that his impatient patients adopted a fix-me-itis attitude that said they wanted to resume their athletic activities promptly, although many were unwilling to accept responsibility for the actions that caused them to seek medical treatment in the first place.

"Stiff joints, aching muscles — many of these 'aging pains' — were actually due to repeated stresses and overuse," Dr. DiNubile said. "Quite often we've found that baby boomers participated in various sport activities years ago as young adults and think they can resume the same activities in their forties and fifties without any modifications."

Another common baby-boomer injury results from years of overuse to the musculoskeletal system: the normal wear and tear of tendons and joints, and muscle loss associated with aging. Many of us are unaware how vulnerable the shoulders and knees are to injury.

Listen up, all you church or office softball team players and rejuvenated tennis players. Just because you played baseball and tennis in high school doesn't mean you can pick up where you left off 25 years ago. And you won't be able to lift weights or pedal a bike as hard as you used to.

No Pain, No Gain? No Way!

"No pain, no gain."

I'm sure you've heard that old bromide as frequently as I have over the years. I always took "no pain, no gain" to mean that I had to be willing to pay the price if I wanted to be successful in an endeavor. If I wanted to become a doctor or a lawyer or pursue some other career, I had to commit to the pain of studying every day of the week and twice on Sunday.

But when it comes to exercise, we need to kill the "no pain, no gain" motto right now and give it a quick burial. That stuff is hooey! Under no circumstances should you create pain while conducting any type of exercise. I'll explain by giving you an example.

Suppose that the first snowstorm of the season — a Nor'easter — dumps two feet of wet, heavy snow on your community. Your driveway and sidewalks must be shoveled before the wet snow melts and turns into an ice rink. You begin pushing and mashing and lifting rock-heavy slabs of snow. After half an hour of strenuous exercise, your body protests — but you're not even halfway finished. You keep shoveling away, doing your best to ignore your aching body.

Your body is aching because during extensive exercise, the muscles (which are made up of small, thread-like muscle fibers) extend and contract. These fibers are arranged in bundles of "cross bridges" of muscle and, under heavy exertion, they break off and become dead tissue. When you woke up with stiffness and soreness the following morning, what you felt were dead muscle cross bridges.

If you looked at those dead muscle tissues with a microscope, those strands of microfibers would resemble spaghetti — not soft, cooked spaghetti, but old, brittle spaghetti strands. When spaghetti comes hot out of the pot, the strands are soft and supple. But if you leave a plate of spaghetti (without any sauce) out overnight, the strands adhere to themselves and cannot be pulled apart. In a day or so, these strands become brittle and easily break into pieces. In a similar way, this is what happens to the body's muscles as we age. Muscle fibers become brittle from lack of use — and then break and cry out in agony when put into action. This is *not* how we want our muscles to react when we exercise.

That's why I preach, throughout this book, about the importance of having a well-balanced training program. Try to incorporate the three pillars of fitness: cardiovascular, strength, and flexibility routines. Regularly stretched muscles will stay toned so that you don't wake up with stiffness and soreness in the morning.

Ways to Avoid Injuries

You may not be able to prevent a sudden muscle pull or back spasm. But that doesn't let you off the hook. You should take prudent steps to *lessen* the chance of injuries visiting your body.

Because exercise is so important to staying healthy, you have to be sensible and take precautions. Look at some ways you can stay out of emergency rooms and doctors' offices.

- ✔ **Always take time to warm up and stretch.** Sure, the ideal warm-up is 15 minutes of easy stretches, followed by ten minutes on the exercise bike. That's not going to happen often, because we don't have the time (or the inclination) to take that long getting loose. A more realistic approach would be stretching and doing a few calisthenics for two to five minutes *before* exercising at the fitness center or warming up for your sport. You should pay attention to stretching the four problem areas for adults: calves, hamstrings, lower back, and the front of the shoulders.

- ✔ **Try to avoid becoming a weekend warrior who compresses a week's worth of athletic activity into one or two days.** Playing in a basketball league on Saturdays, skiing on Sundays, and remaining sedentary the rest of the week sounds like a textbook way to do some serious damage. You've got to work out at least once or twice during the week not including those weekend activities.

✔ **Don't play your sport to get in shape; get in shape to play your sport.** Weekend warriors need to change their mindset regarding *why* they play a sport. You're going to win more matches, score more baskets, drive in more runs, and make more catches when you're in better shape for the games.

✔ **Look for ways to cross-train.** You don't have to be a triathlete to cross-train. Riding a mountain bike or in-line skating occasionally will be a welcome change for a body used to the same form of exercise (such as walking) week in and week out. Cross-training works different muscles and joints, which means that you won't strain muscles that may get overused by one sporting activity.

✔ **If you're jogging or walking, wear good shoes and choose soft terrain.** Although the best sneakers will not prevent injuries, you should still wear relatively new running shoes or sneakers when you're out on the road. (For more on shoes, see Chapter 13.) The choice of terrain is equally important. Walking on dirt paths absorbs some of the impact when the foot contacts the ground. Cement and asphalt are hardest on the body because they cause the entire force of the foot striking the ground to be transmitted to the joints of the feet, ankles, knees, hips, and lower back. If you're walking through a park, gravitate to the grass.

✔ **Wear safety gear.** It's one thing to forget to stretch and limber up before walking or playing tennis, but it's quite another to go in-line skating without a helmet or padding. Adults who ride bicycles die from head injuries at nearly twice the rate as children on bikes, all because many of us figure we don't need a helmet or that helmets are for little kids. The Consumer Product Safety Commission estimates that 69 percent of children wear helmets while biking, while only 43 percent of baby boomers don a "brain bucket." You should set an example for your children — an example that will stay with them all their lives.

✔ **Know that basketball and bicycling cause the most injuries.** Sure, participation counts are higher in these sports, but more than 65,000 bikers and 45,000 basketball players were treated in hospital emergency rooms in 1998.

✔ **Take a lesson every now and then.** If you're an avid golfer (and I know many folks over 40 are crazy about the game), lessons can help you hit the ball properly and avoid lower back problems. The same goes for you tennis players. Many injuries result from bad technique; good instructors can smooth out your swing and help you prevent injuries.

✔ **Make sure that your equipment is in good shape.** Downhill skis should be tuned before each season. Bikes should undergo an annual tune-up. Tennis rackets need to be restrung, lest the string beds become mushy and cause tennis elbow.

✔ **Be willing to use lighter weights.** Just because you always did eight plates on the leg curl machines doesn't mean that your body can handle the same weight mass at age 48. Start with four plates. Maybe after six months of strength training you can work yourself up to eight plates again.

✔ **Use good technique on the weight equipment.** Bench presses, leg presses and extensions, and even arm curls must be performed properly to prevent injuries.

✔ **Don't try to make up for years of inactivity overnight.** You're going to need some time to regain what's been lost. Give your body a chance to recover from a hard workout by doing an easy workout the next time around.

✔ **If you pull a muscle, stop!** Listen to your body. If you are experiencing pain (and by our age, we should know the difference between fatiguing pain and something-went-wrong pain), quit your workout immediately. If you think minor damage has been caused, remember that ice is nice. Go home and ice the tender area. (See the sidebar "Icing's not just for cakes and hockey players.") If you think you did some serious damage, check with a sports medicine professional or your family doctor.

✔ **Remember to give yourself the talk test.** You should be able to talk to a friend while you're exercising (or after finishing). If you're walking with a friend, you should be able to converse normally with her. If you're huffing and puffing, trying to catch your breath, you're walking too fast or need to build up to a longer walking period. The same goes for working out in a fitness center with the cardiovascular equipment (treadmills or stationary bikes) or strength-training machines: You shouldn't exert yourself to the point that you couldn't carry on a conversation with an exercise buddy.

✔ **Finally, admit that you're no longer invulnerable.** Maybe we all need bumper stickers that say, "Injuries happen."

Icing's not just for cakes and hockey players

If you need to ice an injury, do so several times over the first few hours after you get hurt — four to five times for 20 minutes each time. Ice provides pain relief and reduces swelling. Use ice four to five times a day for 20 minutes until the pain abates. You may have to ice for two or three days.

You have a couple of home options for icing down an injury. You can grab a bag of frozen vegetables (corn and peas work great) and put it right on the injured area, or you can fill a Ziploc bag with freezer ice. Be sure to take as much air out of the bag as possible before you set the bag on the injured area. You will probably want to wrap the ice bag in a thin towel so water doesn't leak onto you — or the floor. For those who see themselves icing frequently, you can fill small paper cups with water, freeze them, and use the cups for a much-needed ice massage for muscle soreness. Ice massage also works wonders for working the knots out.

Warning: "Chemical ice" and other rub-on products are ineffective for swelling and inflammation. Ibuprofen, however, is effective but should not be considered a substitute for rest and icing.

You're even vulnerable at work

If you work at a computer for extended amounts of time, you know that you are at risk for various types of repetitive-strain injuries ranging from sore wrists (such as the dreaded carpal tunnel syndrome) to sore necks to sore backs.

Fred Dolan, my friend who developed the StretchMate (see Chapter 15), also serves as the executive director of the American Flexibility Institute. Fred studied computer furniture, and he found that persons who sat before computers for extended periods had difficulty with eye strain and developed shoulder and neck fatigue, as well as back problems.

Fred worked with the National Institute of Occupational Safety and Health (NIOSH) and recommended that employees stretch for 10 minutes after every 60 minutes of work. At first, companies in the testing group balked, but Fred gave the data-entry and word-processing employees a 10-minute stretch routine to follow. Productivity increased by 22 percent, even though the employees worked 10 fewer minutes per hour!

If you are deskbound or have a computer keyboard attached to the end of your fingers all day, stretch and limber up for 5 to 10 minutes every hour. You're going to be more productive to your company, and you're going to be more fitness-friendly to your body. Something you can do at home after a long day of typing is to ice your wrists. This reduces inflammation and provides pain relief.

You don't have to be a white-collar worker to experience wrist problems. You can hit too many tennis balls, which happened in my case. In 1982, I underwent carpal tunnel surgery for the right wrist — my playing hand. The doctor promised me that I would be able to resume my tennis career, and he was right. But when he unwrapped the bandage the day after surgery, the sight of an ugly, 4-inch-long, zig-zag scar along my right wrist caused me to nearly pass out.

Worst-Case Scenario: Signs of Heart Problems

Tweaking an ankle or tipping over on the ski slope is one thing, but feeling heart palpitations, severe constricting pains in the chest, or the dreaded numbness in the left arm is quite another. Those are warning signs of a heart attack.

Heart attacks and cardiovascular disease are more common than you think, which means we need to rethink the image of an overweight guy toppling like a fallen tree. Check this statistic: Cardiovascular diseases, especially coronary heart disease and stroke, are the leading causes of death for *women* in the United States. Heart attacks, strokes, and other cardiovascular diseases have killed more females than males every year since 1984.

The classic symptoms

Let's review the classic symptoms of a heart attack. They include

- A prolonged crushing, squeezing, or burning pain in the center of the chest. The pain may radiate to the neck, one or both arms, or the jaw.
- Uncomfortable pressure or pain in the center of the chest lasting longer than a few minutes.
- Chest discomfort with lightheadedness, fainting, sweating, nausea, or shortness of breath.
- Chills, sweating, and a weak pulse.
- Cold and clammy skin, gray pallor, or a severe appearance of illness.

Less common warning signs include

- Unusual chest, stomach, or abdominal pain.
- Nausea or dizziness.
- Shortness of breath and difficulty breathing.
- Unexplained anxiety, weakness, or fatigue.
- Palpitations, cold sweat, or paleness.

Not all these signs occur in every heart attack. Sometimes, they come and go, which means you have to make a difficult decision: Do you call for help? Do you dial 911 or drive yourself to the emergency room?

Women, beware

Women under 50 were twice as likely as men to die in the hospital after a heart attack, according to a 1999 study published in the *New England Journal of Medicine*. Researchers believe that the crushing chest pain and other warning signs that typify heart attacks are less common for women, which makes their symptoms more difficult to evaluate. For instance, some women experienced subtler symptoms, such as nausea instead of chest pain. (This is not to say that nausea is a precursor to heart attacks for women — just a less common warning sign.)

If your body sends you warning signs, don't excuse them because you don't want to disrupt your plans. Get to a doctor or hospital right away. The life you save *will* be your own.

A disheartening story

On a recent visit to Nick Bollettieri's Tennis Academy in Bradenton, Florida, I asked Adult Tennis Director Chip Brooks how many injuries he sees in the tennis program.

"Daily, weekly, or monthly?" he replied rhetorically.

"Per week," I said.

"We see quite a few injuries," said Chip. "I would say 20 percent of all the adults who come here go down with an injury of some sort — usually muscle pulls or strains."

"Anything serious?"

"Well, let's just say that I'm 0-for-1 with CPR."

"Really?"

"He was 62 years old, an ex-Marine. He was on the tennis court with his group when I noticed he wasn't looking so good. I told him to sit down. It was an uncommonly hot day in March, but he was from Florida, so I figured he was used to the heat. He took a quick break, then walked back to practice his serve.

"He clutched his chest. 'Guys, I think I have a problem,' he said, and boom, he hit the court. Another man started doing mouth-to-mouth, and I did the chest CPR. Paramedics came and shocked him, but he was gone. Later, we heard he died instantly."

A heart attack can take someone's life in the time it takes to read this sentence.

Chapter 19

Keeping Your Cool: Drinking Fluids and Slowing Down

In This Chapter
▶ Staying hydrated
▶ Water and sports drinks: something to quaff about
▶ Taking time to cool down

*N*o doubt about it, this is going to be a "cool" chapter. In it, I tell you about the importance of keeping cool while you exercise (by drinking water or sports drinks) and cooling down *after* your exercise is over.

I will admit that I probably don't drink nearly as many liquids as I should. You may not either, which could be a holdover from your days playing high school sports in the 1960s and '70s. Back then, some coaches thought water breaks were for wimps. Thankfully, that thinking has been discredited as more and more coaches and athletes understand the importance of drinking water — instead of gulping salt tablets — to replace the fluid lost through perspiration. Water has been called the body's most essential nutrient; we can live for weeks without food but just a few days without water. In this chapter, I explain why you shouldn't let your body run low on the water it needs to function properly.

Even if you keep your body hydrated and your throat cool during your workout, you need to end your workout gradually. This chapter explains why suddenly shifting from intense exercise to inactivity shocks your system and wreaks havoc with your circulatory system.

Wetting Your Whistle While You Work Out

For a healthy person, there's no such thing as drinking too much water. On a day-to-day basis, water plays an essential role in maintaining health by

- ✔ Regulating body temperature.
- ✔ Carrying nutrients and oxygen to cells.
- ✔ Cushioning joints.
- ✔ Protecting organs and tissues.
- ✔ Removing toxins.
- ✔ Maintaining strength and endurance.

Your fluid requirements depend on your body weight, lifestyle, age, sex, and the climate in which you live. Younger people need more fluids, as do those in hot climates — no surprise there. I know that I'm more apt to reach for a glass of water after a tennis workout in Orlando than after a taxing ski run in the Colorado Rockies.

You've probably heard that you should drink eight to ten glasses of water each day. That's a *lot* of water. Can that much be drunk? The answer is yes, but you have to work at it.

If you suddenly increase your water intake, you may be wondering where the next toilet can be found. You don't *have* to drink water, however. Those recommended eight glasses can come as other fluids: sports drinks such as Gatorade, fruit juices, milk, and drinks such as Crystal Light. Anything non-caffeinated counts. You also receive significant water from eating fruits and vegetables and even potatoes, cottage cheese, and meat.

Can you drink water and lose weight?

Some people drink as little water as possible, thinking that water will bloat their bodies and keep them from losing weight. Nothing could be further from the truth. Christen Woodland, R.D., performed a study at the University of Utah revealing that participants who had lost three or four pounds through dehydration experienced a 3 percent decrease in how many calories they burned at rest. So the truth is when you don't drink enough fluids, you don't burn as many calories, which means it takes longer for you to lose weight.

The best ways to stay hydrated

If water is good for you while you are not exercising, it's even better for you while you are. During a strenuous workout, your body loses fluids that need replenishing. These fluids perform several crucial functions:

- ✔ Fluids in the blood transport glucose to the muscles that you're working and carry away lactic acid. (Lactic acid builds up when muscles contract vigorously for long periods and the circulatory system falls behind in delivering oxygen to them.)

- ✔ Fluids in urine eliminate waste products from the body.

- ✔ Fluids in sweat dissipate excess heat and cool the body.

If you fail to drink enough fluids or lose too much fluid through sweating, your body goes into the tank, so to speak. Yet most people keep striding away on the treadmill, unaware that they should be sipping on a water bottle every ten minutes or so. The next time you work out, remember these tips regarding proper fluid replacement:

- ✔ The time to start drinking water is *before* your athletic activity, not afterward. Drink a glass or two of water in the hour or two leading up to your workout. This extra fluid will offset sweat losses; any excess will be excreted as urine before you work out. If you're an early morning walker and don't feel like drinking bland water at 6 a.m., drink a glass of orange juice before you walk out the front door. Then grab a water bottle and sip on it while you pace through the neighborhood.

- ✔ While exercising, quaff eight to 16 ounces of water during every 30 minutes of intense exercise — more in hot and humid conditions.

- ✔ If you're working out at a health club, get into the habit of packing a water bottle. Many fitness emporiums are happy to sell you a liter of bottled water for $2. Save the money by bringing your own water, or you can fill up your bottle at the club's drinking fountain, which often dispenses refrigerated water.

- ✔ If, during your match or competition, you have a headache, flushed skin, light-headedness, and a cotton mouth, it's probably too late. Your body has lost too many liquids. You need to drink immediately to stave off the further effects of dehydration, which hampers your performance and can lead to serious health problems, such as heat illness.

- ✔ After finishing your exercise, drink a tall glass of water. Your body is primed to replenish vital fluids that were lost while working out. Slake that thirst right away — before you forget.

What'll you have: Water or a sports drink?

You may be wondering whether you should drink plain water or one of the many sports drinks on supermarket shelves — Gatorade, PowerAde, Allsport, or any other electrolyte cousins.

Water will never go out of style, but Gatorade, in case you haven't noticed, is the 800-pound gorilla in the sports drink market. You see the ubiquitous orange buckets of Gatorade on the sidelines during every major sporting event in the United States, from football, baseball, and basketball to soccer and NASCAR. Gatorade, which commands close to 90 percent of the sports drink market, sells more than 423 million gallons *each day*.

Sports drinks are a mixture of water, a carbohydrate source such as glucose or sugar, and a touch of electrolytes, primarily sodium and potassium. The sodium in sports drinks helps the body retain fluids but encourages you to drink more — which can be a good thing because it keeps you drinking liquids. Gatorade and its sports drink offshoots, however, never leave you feeling as though you've quenched your thirst. Well, it's one way to stay hydrated.

Take a sip of "fitness water"

Just when you think you've seen it all, just when you thought marketeers couldn't come up with something new in "rehydration," you hear news of a new drink: fitness water.

Yes, I said "fitness water." No, this isn't repackaging Evian by slapping a photo of a marathon runner on the plastic bottle. It's an attempt by the makers of Gatorade to create another niche market with a product called Propel.

Propel is your basic H_2O with four B vitamins and two antioxidants (vitamins C and E) added; and it comes in berry, orange, and lemon flavors. Yes, sweeteners have been added, but according to the International Bottled Water Association, if the additives don't add up to more than 1 percent by weight of the final product,

you can still call it water. Because it has only two grams of sugar per serving, Propel slides into home plate and gets a "safe" call.

You might not find Propel everywhere in the United States, but Gatorade hopes to find a buying audience in the women who carry a bottle of Evian with them as they work out on the health club's stair stepper. One appealing factor: The 10 calories per serving is considerably less than Gatorade, which has 50 calories per serving. Both are fat-free.

Propel will probably be very successful, even at $1.25 for a 24-ounce bottle. Gatorade conducted surveys showing that people tend to drink more when a drink is flavored, so they developed Propel for the "active thirst" market.

Sports drinks do offer a competitive advantage by giving you a source of energy during longer activities. The carbohydrates are vital for supplying much-needed energy in long matches or sporting activities lasting more than one hour. But if your exercise consists of striding on a treadmill for 30 minutes or making a quick run-through of strength-training machines, then plain water is fine.

In fact, you'll never go wrong hydrating yourself with tap water or designer water (bottled water you purchase at the store). One drink I cannot recommend is carbonated water like Perrier, although I've seen French tennis players chug that bubbly stuff during changeovers. You really can't improve on fresh, cool water, although Madison Avenue advertising tries hard to convince you otherwise.

Cooling Down after Your Workout

Cooling down does for the end of the workout what stretching and warming up do for the start of one. Believe it or not, cooling down is just as important as limbering up before exercise. The cool-down period is a time for transition from hot-blooded exercise to a gradual slowing of physical activity. If you stop exercising abruptly, blood rushes to the lower extremities, which can cause a dangerous reduction in blood flow to the heart. By slowing down and bringing your exercise time in for a landing, you maintain blood circulation.

Why sudden stops are bad for your body

The goal of exercise is to elevate your heart rate into the target zone of 60 to 80 percent of your maximum heart rate. (See Chapter 6.) Working within this zone gives you maximum health and fat-burning benefits from your fitness activity.

After striding on the treadmill for 40 minutes or playing a spirited game of racquetball, your heart will be pumping nearly twice as fast as its resting rate. Heavy exercise prompts the body to divert blood supply from the internal organs and digestive tract to where it's needed most — usually the legs and arms. The arteries and vessels carrying the blood dilate, or expand, to carry the extra blood coming its way.

After you stop exercising, however, the heart rapidly returns to its normal resting state (unless you're not in the shape you want to be). Because the heart is not pumping as often as it was just a few minutes earlier, blood pressure falls. The dilated arteries and vessels remain larger than normal because they are expecting more blood. When this happens, the body tends to "pool" blood, usually in the legs. With blood pooling around your ankles but little of it reaching the brain, you begin to feel lightheaded from the lack of oxygen. You may feel dizzy and ready to faint. That's why you need to keep moving when you're finished exercising. Cooling down will not prevent muscle soreness, but it will prevent dizziness.

You just need to take a little five-minute walk to elevate your heart rate again. Sure, you could do some stretching as well, but if you're too tired for that, continue to pace about. Walking allows the venous system in your legs to massage the blood upward to the heart, which can then redistribute it to the rest of the body. This also permits the body to rid itself of waste products, such as lactic acid, that cause muscle soreness. If you've ever seen a tennis player cramp at the end of long matches, you've witnessed a player whose body is too tired to pump blood in the volumes needed to flush the body of lactic acid.

Suggestions for ending your workout right

We've talked about taking a five-minute walk to cool down after strenuous exercise. See how this advice plays out with the following scenarios:

✔ You've purchased a new treadmill that's proudly occupying a place in your family room (gotta see that TV). You set the time for 45 minutes and begin walking under the manual mode. After a five-minute warm-up, you dial in your target speed and begin striding briskly.

Cool-down activity: After the 45-minute timer goes off, set a new timer for five minutes, but at a speed considerably slower than what you just finished.

✔ You've rediscovered swimming after all these years out of the pool. Your favorite workout is 30 minutes of lap swimming.

Cool-down activity: Jumping out of the pool with your heart racing is not recommended. Do two more easy laps at half speed, and then get out of the water and walk around the perimeter of the pool before hitting the showers.

✔ You like walking because it's noncompetitive and affords you a stupendous view of the "great outdoors." You're continuing to walk even in the cold winter months.

Cool-down activity: For the last few minutes, walk at a slower pace. The idea is to gradually bring your heart rate down by decreasing the intensity of the workout. If you've been walking around the neighborhood, this might be the time to incorporate some stretching upon your arrival home. You may not be aware of this, but you derive the greatest benefits of stretching when your body is warm, so if you end your walk by immediately sitting down, you're not only wasting an exercise opportunity, but you could wake up the next morning feeling stiff.

✔ You're into strength training these days, eagerly following the routine that your personal trainer has diagrammed for you. You don't waste any time doing the circuit, and you love the "lifting high" that weight machines give you.

Cool-down activity: Ride on a stationary bike for five minutes.

✔ You play in a noontime racquetball league, but you can feel your body losing steam in the second game. Now it's time to go back to the office.

Cool-down activity: For those of you exercising during your lunch hour, you'll have to quit a few minutes early to give yourself time to "walk it off." You won't have enough time to get a good workout *and* cool down properly (by riding a stationary bike, for example), but walking around the club for a few minutes will help. Besides, you can't take a shower right away, or you'll still be sweating when you put your business attire back on!

✔ You split sets on the tennis court and have time for a third. You're sucking wind between points, but you finally pull out the two-hour match in a third-set tiebreaker.

Cool-down activity: Ask your partner to hit a few groundstrokes with you for five minutes. You can also go on a short walk, but don't try to carry your racket bag simultaneously.

✔ After another grueling day on the golf course, you don't know what will give out first: your legs or your electric cart. The "cart path only" rule was a brutal surprise, and now you're wondering if you have enough left in the tank to play the 18th hole.

Cool-down activity: Have a Heineken in the clubhouse bar. Oops! If the golf club has a gym, find a stationary bike. Or ask your partner to drive the cart while you walk the fairways of the last couple of holes.

Part IV
Expanding Your Repertoire

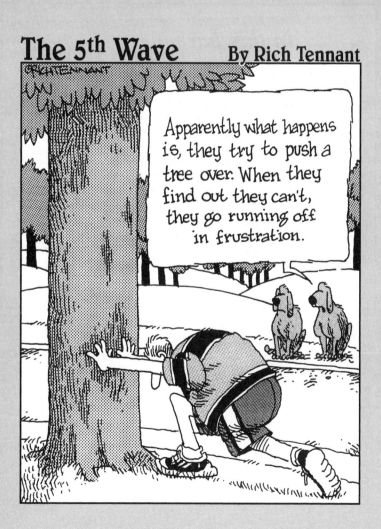

The 5th Wave   By Rich Tennant

Apparently what happens is, they try to push a tree over. When they find out they can't, they go running off in frustration.

In this part . . .

Have a favorite sport? Want to try something new? Then you've come to the right place. This part demonstrates how walking, jogging, tennis, swimming, golfing, bicycling, racquetball, and downhill skiing can fit into your fitness program. But if you're the adventurous sort who wants to try a new athletic experience, then spend time with Chapter 21, where you'll learn about sports that weren't even *invented* in our days of youth — in-line skating, mountain biking, snowboarding, indoor rock climbing, and Tae-Bo. Other fitness trends such as "mind-body" exercises like yoga, tai chi, and Pilates are outlined in Chapter 22. In this part you'll also learn how the nimble fingers of a professional massage therapist can get your blood flowing and work out kinks in your muscles.

Chapter 20

How Your Favorite Sports and Activities Fit into Your Fitness Program

*Y*ou don't have to pump away on a futuristic-looking stair stepper to get your exercise jones. You don't have to sign up for a cardio-kickboxing class to raise your heart rate. You don't even have to lift anything heavier than a five-pound dumbbell to get strong.

This doesn't mean that you should give up these healthy activities. Not at all. What I'm saying is that participating in your favorite sport or physical activity — or taking up something new that looks fun — can become your *main* route to becoming physically fitter in your forties. If you play tennis, swim laps, shoot hoops, or walk miles throughout your neighborhood several times a week, using a stair climber or joining an aerobics class is just the proverbial icing on the fitness cake. (It would still be a good idea to do some weight training, however, for reasons that I explain in Chapter 6.)

You can use any number of sports or physical activities to get in shape and stay in shape. Pick one that will challenge your heart and develop your muscles.

Pick one that will be *enjoyable* for you. Isn't the fun factor what attracted you to play sports when you were younger?

Wondrous Walking

"It is better to walk than to run," says a Hindu proverb, and that's good fitness advice, too. Walking is probably the most perfect exercise you can do and is a surprisingly effective strategy for long-term health. Walking doesn't cost a cent (unless you walk on a treadmill), can be done at any time, is not injurious, and can be as intensive as you want it to be. This load-bearing exercise places a gentle strain on the hips and the rest of the body.

The upside: Benefits almost too numerous to mention

Allow me to rhapsodize in greater detail about this superb, all-around form of fitness:

- **Walking gently exercises all parts of the body in a steady rhythm, gradually imposing mild stress on the heart.** This mild stress makes the heart work harder, builds up heart muscle, and builds a fail-safe collateral circulation system that provides another way to bring blood to the heart if a clot or blockage occurs.

- **Walking can be done at any time you want.** You can get up and go during dawn patrol, forgo the morning coffee break for a walk around the industrial park, walk on your lunch hour, jump on a treadmill after work, or watch the sun set in the west during an after-dinner stroll.

- **You go at your own pace.** You decide how much you want to put into this exercise.

- **You can walk every day.** Unlike strength training and hard jogging, where the muscles need 24 to 48 hours to recoup, walking is an exercise that can be done every day.

- **You can walk after eating.** No one feels like jogging, running around the tennis court, or playing in a senior basketball league on a full stomach. But you can walk after any meal.

- **Walking is a great social exercise.** Because you're not panting from exertion, you can carry along a civilized conversation with a friend or loved one as you stride down the sidewalk or through the picturesque countryside.

- **You don't mess up your hairdo by getting all sweaty.** When the temperature is cool or cold, you rarely perspire unless you're power walking.

Not getting all sweaty is another reason why walking is a favored work-time exercise: You can walk during your break without having to shower and blow-dry your hair afterward.

- **Walking is a sport both sexes can do.** Strength and size don't count for much when walking.

- **Walking can jump-start your day.** If you feel stiff and lethargic upon waking up (and who doesn't these days?), taking a five-minute walk right away will wake up your nervous system. If you're fighting early morning lethargy, stick your feet in a bucket of ice water and then go on a walk, something that's sure to get you going.

- **Walking can be done in the privacy of your home.** Many people prefer to do their walking on a treadmill, which I heartily approve of because I use our treadmill for that purpose. If it's cold or rainy or dark outside — or if you don't feel safe walking in your neighborhood after hours — step on a treadmill.

- **Walking gives you time to think.** We're so rushed these days, who has time to think things through? Walking is a welcome respite from our 500-channel, ten-phone-messages, tons-of-e-mail existence that assaults our senses each day.

The downside: Short and sweet

You have to go the extra mile to find anything bad about walking. The worst thing you can say is that you need plenty of time to walk up a head of steam. Substantial health benefits don't start appearing until you walk several times a week for about an hour each time. Some people also find walking too boring for their taste, while others complain that walking doesn't deliver a hardcore workout. Those are minor quibbles in my book, however.

Getting started: Betsy's one-month walking plan

Walking is a form of exercise in which you choose the pace, but you'll greatly help your overall fitness if you follow a proven walking program. If you're ready to choose walking as your exercise, you need to be aware that the President's Council on Physical Fitness and Sports has designated three walking speeds:

- Slow, or 3 mph
- Brisk, or 4 mph
- Fast, or 4.5 mph

Table 20-1 indicates how fast it takes to walk a few specific distances at each of these speeds. After you know how far you are walking and the pace you want to keep, you can set a target time.

Table 20-1	Time (in Minutes) for Various Distances		
Distance	*Slow walk (3 mph)*	*Brisk walk (4 mph)*	*Fast walk (4.5 mph)*
0.5 mile	10:00	7:30	6:40
1 mile	20:00	15:00	13:20
1.5 miles	30:00	22:30	20:00
2 miles	40:00	30:00	26:40
2.5 miles	50:00	37:30	33:20
3 miles	60:00	45:00	40:00
3.5 miles	70:00	52:30	46:40
4 miles	80:00	60:00	53:20
4.5 miles	90:00	67:30	60:00
5 miles	100:00	75:00	66:40

Note: Most people 40 and up cannot keep up a "fast" pace while walking, but it's a goal to shoot for.

Time yourself for a half-hour walk through your neighborhood, then drive the same route in your car to measure how far you walked. With that information, you will get a good idea of how to pace yourself when following this walking plan:

First Week

Day 1	Walk 1 mile slowly (at 3 mph pace)
Day 2	Walk 1 mile slowly
Day 3	Walk 1.5 miles slowly
Day 4	Walk 1.5 miles slowly
Day 5	Walk 2 miles slowly
Day 6	Walk 2 miles slowly
Day 7	Rest

Second Week

Day 1	Walk 2.5 miles slowly
Day 2	Walk 2.5 miles slowly
Day 3	Walk 3 miles slowly
Day 4	Walk 3 miles slowly
Day 5	Walk 3.5 miles slowly
Day 6	Walk 3.5 miles slowly
Day 7	Rest

Third Week

Day 1	Walk 4 miles slowly
Day 2	Walk 2 miles briskly (at 4 mph pace)
Day 3	Walk 4 miles slowly
Day 4	Walk 2.5 miles briskly
Day 5	Walk 4 miles slowly
Day 6	Walk 3 miles briskly
Day 7	Rest

Fourth Week

Day 1	Walk 4.5 miles slowly
Day 2	Walk 3.5 miles briskly
Day 3	Walk 5 miles slowly
Day 4	Walk 4 miles briskly
Day 5	Walk 5 miles slowly
Day 6	Walk 4.5 miles briskly
Day 7	Rest

After two weeks of walking, your blood pressure begins to drop. In weeks three and four, cholesterol counts fall (unless you're eating puffed cheese snacks while you walk). With a couple of months under your belt, your heart and lungs become stronger and work more efficiently. Your resting pulse decreases, and your bones become stronger. You can even expect to lose a pound or two with each month of walking.

You're going to find yourself in super shape after following a walking regimen. A rosy-apple glow will reappear in your cheeks, the fruit of a fresh sense of well-being. Your body will have a new foundation for fitness that you can call upon if you pursue other athletic endeavors, such as playing on a softball team, snow skiing in the Rockies, or joining a tennis league.

Improve that posture

Walking is a superlative way to work on your posture. Ask your walking partner if your walking posture is hunched over. Straighten up. Breathe deep. Then lean slightly forward from the ankles, not the waist, and walk straight ahead with purpose. Your posture will improve.

Swinging the arms while walking turns the exercise into a total body activity. Keep your elbows bent at a 90-degree angle, and swing from the shoulder. Your hand should end its forward swing at breastbone height. As for striding, keep everything long and smooth. The foot on the ground should stay there as long as possible before pushing off.

Too cold to walk?

You don't have any excuse for not starting a walking program if you live near a mall (and there're only about 2,400 shopping malls dotting the landscape of our country). Malls are great places to walk because of the hospitable temperature-controlled environment and engaging window displays along the way. Many malls have walking clubs and open their doors from 6:30 to 10 a.m. so walkers can have the run of the place before the stores open.

Running to Fitness

Running or jogging (I use the terms interchangeably) can be hard on the body's muscles and joints, especially the knees and back. Most people over the age of 40, I believe, would rather walk away from running, and I understand the rationale. Running is not easy and requires discipline. At our age, we're better off playing an enjoyable sport, walking, or using fitness machines to become fit, which is why I contend that running in the forties, fifties, and sixties is best left to lifelong adherents to this form of exercise.

A rundown of running's benefits

Now that I've dissed jogging, let me point out some of the positive aspects of this demanding physical activity:

- **Like walking, you can jog anytime and anywhere.** You don't need a buddy, and you don't need lots of equipment. Proper clothes and good running shoes are enough.

✔ **Jogging delivers the same benefits as walking — only faster.** Running improves muscle tone and strength, relieves stress, and combats osteoporosis, heart disease, and arthritis.

✔ **Running burns plenty of calories, especially for intense road workouts.** A half-hour jog burns around 750 calories, a lot for a short time. A jogging workout is a very efficient way to achieve cardiovascular fitness.

✔ **Jogging is a great exercise for business travelers.** Finding convenient fitness centers on the road can be difficult, and they are expensive. You can jog from your hotel when you have a break in your schedule.

✔ **You experience a "runner's high."** Something can be said for how good you feel after a good run when endorphins are released by the body into the bloodstream.

Running can take a toll on the body

Why is running, which is such a simple exercise, so hard to do? Because running is *strenuous*. Running in our middle-age years requires intense effort, quickly saps our dwindling energy, and is not kind to aging joints in the knees and hips. The back muscles protest each jolting stride on the pavement. Simply put, jogging jars the body.

TIP

Stay safe!

We have all heard the all-too-familiar news reports of joggers and walkers being hit by cars or suddenly ambushed by strangers intent on doing harm. Even if you live in a safe neighborhood, please take the following precautions to stay out of harm's way while you're running (or walking):

✔ Invite a friend along. Two is always better than one.

✔ Lock your house and take a key with you. Someone may be casing your place.

✔ Stick to areas you know. When you're on a jog, this is not the time to go exploring.

✔ Avoid going out after dark, if possible. If not, stay on lighted streets.

✔ Consider running or walking indoors. Many cold-weather fitness clubs have elevated tracks that ring the inside perimeter of the building.

✔ Go against traffic. Assume that you don't have the right-of-way.

✔ Wear bright colors so drivers can see you. Even glow-in-the-dark shoes can help.

✔ Stay away from bushy areas where someone could hide.

✔ Carry a Mace-type or pepper spray with you.

✔ If followed, go to the nearest house or business and call 911.

✔ If someone looks like he's going to attack you, yell your head off.

Running can also be a bit dangerous if you don't live in a pedestrian-friendly town. A lack of sidewalks means that you find yourself sharing the road with cars and bicycles, and cars and bikes win every time. And jogging on uneven road shoulders can make ankle or leg problems worse — another reason why joint injuries are common among runners.

Getting started around the track

If jogging is something you want to do, however, be my guest. If you're picking it up after a long layoff — or even if you're a first-time jogger — following these steps can help get you on your way:

1. **Get good running shoes.** Jogging in a pair of no-support Keds or well-worn tennis shoes is inviting trouble. You can't go wrong purchasing running shoes made for the market by Nike, New Balance, Reebok, and so on. Check for fit, cushioning of the heel, and arch support. Be sure to have the shoe salesperson measure your foot width.

   New Balance sells running shoes in various widths.

2. **Start out by walking and then jogging a little bit.** Walk and jog. Walk and jog. I hate to break the news to you, but at our age, we're probably not going to be able to jog nonstop for the first week or two.

3. **When you are up and running, jog for at least 30 minutes.** The first five to ten minutes of any jog are given to working out age-related kinks until the juices start flowing. If you stop at the ten-minute mark, you haven't moved a step along the path of physical fitness. Thirty minutes is minimum; 40 minutes are better.

4. **Don't worry about the distance covered.** Just keep plugging away for the time you've set aside to jog.

5. **Run for two days, and then take a rest.** Taking a rest is mandatory, because recovery is a part of training. The optimal schedule is running at least four days a week, with days of rest included in that week.

Tennis, Anyone?

Can I put a plug in for this sport of a lifetime that has been so good to me? Tennis consists of quick, almost savage-like action followed by relatively tranquil intervals. This fiercely competitive game is a marvelous activity filled with great mental stimulation. The best thing I can say about tennis is that you'll never get bored playing it. No matter what your level, you'll see an improvement every time you step on the court.

A game set up to match your fitness needs

Although tennis cannot be strictly considered as an aerobic sport, I must point out that it's a game requiring stamina, running, and strength. If you play singles with an evenly matched opponent, you'll get all the workout you want. Most players in the forties and up, however, play doubles, which is less exercise because you have to cover only half the court. But playing two or three sets of doubles packs plenty of exercise, which is why tennis is a popular sport for us senior players.

Tennis works your body in unexpected ways. The game builds nearly every muscle group, especially those in your legs and arms. You develop flexibility because you have to stay low and keep your knees bent when you hit forehands and backhands. Rapid twists and turns work the muscles of the lower body, including the buttocks, front of the thigh, and calf muscles. And serving is a complicated process that involves dozens of muscles in a full range of motion.

The better you get at tennis, the more you run — as long as you're matched with an opponent who can keep a rally going. In tennis, you run from side to side, up to the net and back, and chase lobs struck by your diabolical adversary. When the ball is in play, you keep making small, mincing steps in between shots, so you're constantly moving until the point is over.

And then you rest — but not for long. Tennis is a game of short bursts of muscular activity followed by brief periods of rest. A well-played game places significant demands on your cardiovascular system.

No, tennis isn't for everyone

Pitty-pat tennis between beginners involves little exercise, so you have to have some skill before you can access tennis's full fitness benefits. This is easier said than done because tennis is a difficult game to master; nobody knows that better than I. The game's long learning curve requires hours of practicing the proper strokes, as well as studying the game's finer points.

You can get injured playing tennis. Players of any age can twist an ankle making a sudden change in direction, and older players complain of stiff backs, sore shoulders, and arthritic knees. If you learn to hit the ball incorrectly, you run the risk of developing tennis elbow, which feels like someone is jabbing a small needle into your elbow area each time you strike the ball.

While the U.S. has thousands of public courts that anyone can play on, those living in four-season climates must pay through the nose to play indoors during the late fall, winter, and early spring months. The cost of tennis balls hasn't changed much in 20 years, but $295 for a titanium-braided frame racket seems a bit much for recreational use.

Burn those calories playing tennis — and other sports as well

Here are the amounts of calories burned in three hours of exercise per week:

Sport	Calories burned
Tennis (competitive)	1,934
Aerobics (moderate)	1,704
Tennis (moderate)	1,602
In-line skating (moderate)	1,397
Downhill skiing (moderate)	1,387
Basketball (moderate)	1,280
Cycling (10 mph)	1,268
Weightlifting	1,204
Baseball	1,032
Walking (15-minute mile)	909
Tennis (casual)	860
Golf (walking with hand cart)	860
Fishing	645
Housework (moderate)	645

Source: GE Sports Science

Getting started: Leave it to the pros

If you're new to the game, you have to seek out private professional instruction. A certified pro can teach you how to properly make the forehand and backhand strokes and serve and volley motions correctly. Each stroke is different, and there are various grip changes to learn. Let a good pro show you how to play tennis, and you'll enjoy the game much more — and get a much better on-court workout.

Look for pros certified by the U.S. Professional Tennis Association (USPTA). They are usually found at tennis clubs and, to a lesser extent, health clubs with tennis courts. Word of mouth counts for a lot as well, so ask around. Tennis players will tell you who does the best job teaching you how to play.

Most tennis courts are what we call *hardcourts* (an asphalt or concrete surface topped with a special paint). Hardcourts are hard on the knees and back, however. Try to find a club with "soft" courts, or playing surfaces made of green clay-like composition. Called Har-Tru or Lee Fast-Dri, these clay courts are so easy on the body that you'll be able to play a best-of-five-set match with your doubles buddies.

Hardcourts, which are cheaper to build and maintain than clay courts, are found at municipal parks, high schools, and nearly all private and public tennis clubs west of the Rockies. You can find soft courts at private clubs in Texas, throughout the Southeast, and along the Atlantic Seaboard. If you play tennis more than once a week, it may be worth it to join a club with clay courts.

Swimming in Exercise

If you don't like getting sweaty while you exercise, want to take a load off your weight-bearing joints, and just love being in water, then swimming could be your sport.

Jump on in, the water's great

Water has an irresistible appeal. Its magical qualities are readily apparent from the moment you jump in; the upward force of water buoys you and diminishes the downward pull of gravity. This phenomenon results in less stress on load-bearing joints like the knees and hips and, therefore, fewer injuries. The only way you can get hurt would be swimming straight into the pool wall or jumping into water that's shallower than you are expecting.

Water supports you, adds natural resistance that tones and strengthens the body's muscles, and works your muscles in the same way that light weights do. Water creates buoyancy that reduces the effects of gravity by 90 percent, allowing you to exercise with minimal impact on your joints. The pressure of water against your chest works your lungs and improves the body's respiratory system. Another thing I like about swimming is that you don't have to be any good at it to benefit from its aerobic-inducing qualities. You can dog paddle up and down the swimming lanes and still receive a workout that leaves you panting.

If you're monitoring your heart as a swimmer, realize that your target heart rate will be around 13 beats per minute *slower* than with any other exercises. This is because you are usually in the prone position while swimming, and your body is submerged in a cool environment. But you don't have to swim longer to get the same cardiovascular workout as you would in other sports.

Swimming is also great exercise for those rehabbing from a sports injury or minor surgery. Around five years ago when I had serious knee surgery, I was required to be non–weight-bearing for three months, which meant crutches and even a wheelchair on occasion. Swimming became my fitness savior, and that's when I became a great fan of aquatic exercises. Swimming can keep your fitness up until you're able to get back to your usual weight-bearing sport, such as walking or skiing.

You can use several swimming strokes (and you may have learned a couple of these in swim classes long ago). The propulsive power in these arms-and-legs motions benefits the muscles in those areas. The better your stroke technique, the more efficient your swimming workouts become. You'll be able to swim faster and longer, instead of flailing away at the water.

Let's take a closer look at the well-known swimming strokes:

- **Freestyle:** Alternate overarm strokes and up-and-down kicks.

- **Sidestroke:** While turned on your side, do a *scissors kick* (open and close your legs like scissors) as you reach out with a sidearm stroke.

- **Butterfly:** Of all the strokes, the butterfly is by far the most difficult to learn. You start by learning to undulate your body. Your arms begin in front of your shoulders; then you flex your hands down and push them to the outside to create lift. You continue undulating while your legs perform a *dolphin kick,* which is a feet-together kick.

- **Breaststroke:** In this stroke, your arms and legs move together. Just under the surface of the water, your arms perform a forward circular pull while your legs do a scissors kick. As with the butterfly, you should have a professional swim coach teach you how to perform these complicated strokes.

- **Backstroke:** While lying on your back, reach back with an alternating overarm stroke, kicking simultaneously. My daughter, Maggie, has been taking swim lessons, and Shannon, her instructor, told her to "reach up and pretend you're picking apples."

Pick a stroke — any stroke — and dive right in. The water should be just right.

The drawbacks of swimming

Although I've never been an avid swimmer, I've swum plenty of laps over the years. I admire those who can shut off the outside world and concentrate on the black striping on the bottom of the pool while they stroke and kick from one end to another. Even swimmers have to admit there isn't much to look at while they train, unlike joggers and bicyclists, who can enjoy the outdoor scenery as they pump their legs.

Other drawbacks include:

- ✔ Swimming isn't a weight-bearing exercise, so swimming laps won't prevent osteoporosis.

- ✔ Unless you have your own pool, you're limited to swimming at certain hours in public facilities. Many neighborhoods have community pools these days, but they're drained during the winter months.

- ✔ Swimmers are guaranteed wet hair dripping with chlorine, which can dry and dull hair (which is why you don't see too many swimming aficionados with long hair these days).

Overexertion is common among swimming neophytes who dive into the pool and begin thrashing away, arms and legs churning like a Mississippi steamboat. If you haven't swum in years but think you can pick up where you left off 35 years ago when you won the peewee division at a summer swim meet, guess again. Take it easy! Warm up by stretching *before* you jump in the pool, and then swim two or three easy laps before taking stock of your fitness. You may want to call it a day right there, which is fine. Tomorrow, swim three more laps.

You don't need to swim laps to benefit

You certainly don't have to swim laps to get a water workout. The following exercises can be done in the shallow end of the pool:

Toe raises

Toe raises are a good exercise to start with. Stand next to the pool wall and hold the edge with your feet shoulder-width apart. Rise up on the balls of your feet and hold for a count of four. Relax for a few seconds, and then stand on your toes again for a count of four. Do a set of ten.

Benefits: This exercise makes your calf muscles stronger.

Leg curls

To do leg curls, turn sideways to the pool wall and hold the edge with your left hand, feet shoulder-width apart. Bend your right leg as far as you can; then reach down with your right hand and bring your right foot to your right buttock. Stretch to a count of five. Do a set of six, and then turn and repeat the exercise with your left leg.

Benefits: Leg curls stretch your quadriceps and work your hip joints and lower back.

Lunges

Start the lunge exercise by placing both hands on your hips in shallow water. Step forward with your right leg as far as you can, and then hold the step for a count of six. Straighten up to a standing position. Now step forward with your left leg as far as you can. Hold the step for count of six. Repeat 12 times.

Benefits: This exercise stretches your hamstrings and leg muscles while working the knees.

Arm circles

This exercise requires that you move to deeper water, about neck height. In the deeper water, stretch out both of your arms and make tiny circles in a clockwise direction. Count to 20; then rest. Repeat this step six times. Next make arm circles in a counterclockwise direction to a count of 20; rest. Repeat the counterclockwise six times as well.

Benefits: The arm-circle exercise firms up your shoulders and upper arms.

Pull-Ups

If your pool has a small diving board, you can do a water version of the pull-up. Jump up and grab end of the diving board. Pull yourself up, much like chin-ups in the school yard. Repeat 12 times.

Benefits: Pull-ups strengthen your upper back and arms.

Running from side to side

If you think getting out of quicksand would be difficult, wait until you try running in the shallow end. Start at one side of the pool in the shallow end and then run to the other side of the shallow end. Keep your legs churning. Rest. When you're ready to go again, take off for the other side. Do this ten times or until you're no longer capable.

Benefits: This is a great aerobic exercise that strengthens the legs.

Teeing It Up

"Golf is a good walk spoiled," said Mark Twain, but I'm afraid that golf isn't even a good walk. To gain the cardiovascular benefits of walking, you need to move continuously for at least 20 minutes with no stopping to hit golf balls, look for errant shots, take two whacks in the bunker, or properly line up that all-important fourth putt. No, golf needs to be viewed as a supplement to your daily fitness routine.

It may not be a good walk, but it is a walk of sorts

We can, of course, ascribe *some* physical good to walking 7,200 yards when playing from the blue tees. So walking in golf is always going to be better than *not* walking. But this means you should leave the cart behind at the pro shop whenever you can. For those courses where cart rentals are mandatory, periodically ask your buddy if you can walk to your next shot while he drives.

A pulled muscle waiting to happen

Around two-thirds of the golfing population suffers some type of golf-related injury after the age of 50, usually sprains and muscle pulls. Many golfers drive into the parking lot, open up the car trunk, put on their golf shoes, and heft their heavy bags to the pro shop. Within minutes, they're standing on the first tee, their No. 1 drivers in hand.

"You're up," says your usual Saturday morning golf buddy. A couple of practice swings and you give your oversized, bubble-shafted, titanium-juiced driver a full whirl and toe the ball into the adjoining fairway. You feel a twinge in your lower back.

"I think I'll take a mulligan," you say, as you re-tee a ball. Two more practice swings, and then you coil and unload once again, only to see your second ball join the first. This time your back *really* hurts.

That's golf: a sport of truncated warm-ups, pulled muscles, and sore backs. To reduce your chance of injury, warm up *before* you drive to the golf club. Fifteen minutes on the treadmill or stationary bike, a brisk walk around the block, and some easy calisthenics (arm circles, jumping jacks, and lunges) help loosen up the muscles. And after you get to the golf course, give yourself at least 15 minutes to warm up before heading to the first tee.

Getting ready to use the sticks

Nearly every golf course has a driving range. Take a small bucket of balls and perform the following exercises to prepare for your round:

- ✔ **Step sideways.** Step your right foot out and back, and then your left foot out and back. Repeat several times.

- ✔ **Arm swings.** Keep your arms straight as you slowly cross them in front of you. Spread your shoulder blades apart; then slowly swing your arms out to the side while squeezing your shoulder blades together. Do this six to 12 times.

✔ **Stretch the trunk, shoulders, and hamstring and calf muscles.** Place an iron behind your back and through your arms, and then swivel from side to side for 30 seconds. Turn the other direction and swivel for another 30 seconds.

✔ **Swing two clubs.** Take two irons and make short chipping-like swings to loosen the muscles. Gradually make the swings longer and longer. Following this, take some easy full swings with just one club.

✔ **Start with wedges.** When you're ready to hit, use your pitching iron or loft wedges, which use shorter swings. Because the driver, 3 wood, and 5 wood involve the full swing, don't practice your woods until you're good and warm.

If you don't have time to warm up on the driving range, the following stretching exercises are better than nothing:

✔ **Low back stretch.** Sit with good posture on a bench or golf-cart seat. Keep your feet on the floor. Slowly turn to the right to the point of mild tension. Hold this pose for several seconds, and then repeat on the left side. Do this a half-dozen times.

✔ **Hip stretch.** Sit and cross your right leg over the left with the right ankle resting on the left knee. Lean forward and feel the lower back stretch. Hold this pose several times for five seconds; then repeat with your left ankle over your right knee.

✔ **Hamstring stretch.** Stand next to a bench or the golf cart. Extend your left leg until it's straight on the bench or golf cart seat. Keep your back straight and chin up as you slowly lean forward. Hold this position for several seconds, and then repeat with your right leg.

✔ **Shoulder and arm stretch.** Grab the end of your driver with your right hand and hold the club behind your head with the grip pointing toward the ground. Let your left hand reach behind your back and hold the club as far up the shaft as you comfortably can. Stretch and hold this position for several seconds; repeat with your left hand holding the club head.

✔ **Chest and shoulder stretch.** Hold the golf club horizontally behind your back with both hands, palms facing out. Slowly raise your arms until you feel a mild stretch in your chest and shoulders. Keep a good posture and don't lean forward.

✔ **Side bend stretch.** Hold a golf club horizontally above your head with both hands. Slowly lean to the right until you feel a mild stretch on the left side of your trunk. Hold this pose for several seconds, and then repeat by leaning to the left side.

When the tee is open, don't volunteer to be the first in your foursome to tee off. Let the others go while you take practice swing after practice swing. Try to get in 12 to 15 swings before you tee it up for keeps. Then grip it and rip it!

Tiger prowls the workout room first

One of my neighbors is a golfer named Tiger Woods. Perhaps you've heard of him. Number-one player in the world. Longest hitter. Best putter. Brings his "A game" to nearly every tournament he enters.

Tiger is a tremendously fit athlete: I've seen him jog in the neighborhood, and I know that he works out ferociously in the Isleworth fitness center. His whippet body is *strong*, and he's developed rock-hard, chiseled abs that infomercial companies would die for.

Tiger didn't get buff playing golf, however, which leads me to this point: Golf is nothing more than a long stroll in the park, exercisewise. And if you're riding in a cart (which most golfers do, and most courses demand these days), you can get more exercise doing the grocery shopping. That's why there's a move afoot (so to speak) to get golfers to walk more. The United States Golf Association (USGA), to paraphrase golf teaching legend Harvey Penick, has taken dead aim at the 1,000 U.S. golf courses with a mandatory-use policy regarding golf carts.

"We strongly believe that walking is the most enjoyable way to play golf and that the use of carts is detrimental to the game," said David Fay, the USGA's executive director. "This negative trend needs to be stopped now before it becomes accepted that riding in a cart is the way to play golf."

Amen.

Golf course owners contend that mandatory carts speed up play, but everyone knows the real reason is that carts boost revenue, pure and simple. The USGA is so fired up about the walking issue that it has produced a free informative booklet for USGA members titled *Call to Feet: Golf Is a Walking Game*. Call the USGA headquarters in Far Hills, New Jersey, at (800) 223-0041 to receive your copy.

Get fit to play golf — not vice versa

Many out-of-shape golfers run out of energy on the back nine and the wheels come off in a flurry of double and triple bogeys. Getting fit will help you finish strong, and I know how much you golfers are always looking for ways to shave a few strokes off your handicaps (I'm married to a certified golf nut named Mark McCormack). Golfers who enhance their physical fitness and stretching capabilities see a 5 percent increase in their clubhead speed. Translation: The fitter you are, the farther you're going to hit the ball.

Take a Bike!

One thing you can say about riding a bike: You never forget how to pedal and keep your balance. So biking is an athletic activity that you can pick up all over again. Outdoor cycling is a popular exercise; today's streamlined road bikes efficiently churn up the miles and allow you to burn calories like an incinerator. You can pedal at a moderate pace, or drop a gear and really crank it up.

This section deals with riding road bikes on paved roads and bike trails. In Chapter 21, I talk about mountain bike riding on backcountry trails and "off road." Whatever form of bike riding you choose, the fact remains that this athletic activity represents one of the most perfect matches between the human body and the machine. When you seat yourself on a lightweight, multispeed bicycle and quickly self-generate a fantastic rate of speed, you are part of a modern-day marvel.

If you last rode a bike during your freshman year of college, you'll be amazed at what technology has wrought. Today's road bikes are made of superlight materials, the wheels are thinner than ever, and even the seat technology has improved to the point that you shouldn't be saddle sore the next day.

Burn, baby, burn: Melting those calories

No one has ever cast doubt on the efficacy of biking. Cycling for a half-hour a day burns the equivalent of 11 pounds a year, according to the Bicycle Commuting for Health and Fitness report. Besides the caloric torch-fest that goes on within your body, biking builds leg strength, endurance, and lung power.

No one will argue the point that bicycling is easier on your body than running. Cycling is friendly to the joints, which is important for middle-aged exercisers. As you get older, your muscles can still take a lot of work, but your knees, hips, and shoulders cannot endure as much pounding.

Don't just spin your wheels

Cycling won't help you, however, while you're coasting downhill or waiting for the stoplight to turn green. You have to keep the pedal cadence up if you want an aerobic workout. If you find yourself pedaling leisurely just to enjoy the sights, you may need to find a type of exercise that forces you to keep your nose to the grindstone.

Cycling's drawbacks are few. You can get a sore neck from having to hold it up during a long ride, and sharing busy thoroughfares with Mack trucks is not for the faint of heart. You shouldn't ride at night, even if you're wearing reflective clothing and have the right lighting; you can't spot upcoming potholes or rocks in the road. If you lose control and hit the pavement, road rash *hurts*.

The two-wheel commute: Fitting a bicycling workout into your busy day

Commuting to work on a bike not only guarantees five days of weekly exercise, but helps ease rush hour traffic jams and boosts the environment as well. Bike commuting, in this era of rising gas prices, can save you buckets of money (operating an automobile costs about 40 cents a mile). In addition, riding a bike may even be a *faster* way to work than waiting in line on the expressway.

Yet for all its plus marks, bicycle commuting has several daunting problems to hurdle:

- ✔ **Meteorological elements.** Whether you live in rain-soaked Seattle or hot and humid Houston, you may arrive at work looking like a drowned puppy or an exhausted marathon runner. To do the commute, your place of business must have shower facilities.

- ✔ **Environmental elements.** Bikers share asphalt and concrete roadway with two-ton SUVs piloted by distracted mothers and snappy sedans driven by white-collar workers. In this mismatch, heavy metal always trumps flesh and blood.

- ✔ **Time elements.** Because most bike commutes are between 30 and 60 minutes each way, you have to budget enough time to ride to work, shower, and change into new clothes.

- ✔ **Hassle elements.** You can't bring along a pressed pantsuit or coat-and-jacket ensemble when you ride, which means that proper business attire has to be waiting for you upon your arrival. Then you need toiletries for the shower, time to blow-dry your hair, and some new biking clothes to change into for the commute home.

My intention is not to throw a wet poncho over bike riding, but to remind you that these obstacles must be overcome.

Bike commuting will work for you if:

- ✔ **Your place of business has shower facilities.** You have to be able to change out of soaked or sweaty clothes.

- ✔ **You live within a reasonable distance of work.** If you live ten or 15 minutes from work, bike commuting will work easily. If you have a longer ride, look at bike commuting as your aerobic exercise that day.

- ✔ **You don't have to be anywhere quickly after work ends.** If you're rushing home to see a child's ballgame or pick her up from piano lessons, bike commuting won't work.

- ✔ **You feel confident contending with cars and trucks.** You can increase your safety by using a bike trail — if one exists — during your commute.

Time for Racquetball

If you're looking for invigorating exercise, then racquetball is your sport. Marked by short spurts of running and quick changes of direction, racquetball delivers a fast-paced, intense workout.

Racquetball beats the stationary machines

Racquetball burns more calories per hour than a stair stepper or stationary bike. Racquetball players rev up to a constant 75 percent to 85 percent of their maximum heart rate and work nearly every muscle group. The off-the-wall game is lively, the ball flies all over the place, and you can always mount a comeback because there's no clock. Quick reactions and hustle are more important than sheer athleticism.

And racquetball is the easiest racket sport to play, requiring little skill to pick up a racket that looks like a snowshoe and squarely hit the lively rubber ball. There's no net to hit over, either — just smack the ball as hard as you can toward the front wall. Playing the hollow blue ball as it ricochets off the 20-foot walls or comes off the back wall is a challenge, however, and kill shots take great skill. Scoring is easy: If the server wins the rally, he gets a point; the non-server is fighting for the right to serve. Most games are played to 15 points, two-out-of-three takes. The rubber game is an 11-point tiebreaker.

A young man's game?

Racquetball seems to have plateaued in popularity in the last 15 years. Young legs dominate the racquetball population: Two-thirds of the players, predominantly male, are between the ages of 18 and 34. The sport must be played indoors at fitness clubs, and popular reservation times (5 to 7 p.m.) can be hard to come by.

Racquetball can be a dangerous sport because of the close proximity of the two combatants (or four, if you're crazy enough to play doubles). Players get wrapped up in the tight quarters and turn ankles. The walls can be rather unforgiving. Tennis elbow is a possibility. You risk losing an eye from an errant shot or someone's follow-through, unless you wear safety goggles. Those who fail to warm up tear muscles.

But don't let any of that stop you from playing racquetball!

Finding a place to play

Racquetball courts are found at fitness clubs, and the larger the club, the more likely it will have a gleaming racquetball court or two for its members. Often, however, fitness clubs charge extra to play racquetball — usually $10 per person for an hour-long reservation. An active club will organize "challenge ladders" pitting players of equal ability, but the rest of the time, it's up to you to find your own game.

If you're new to racquetball, it's a good idea to take several lessons because playing balls off the walls takes some getting used to. The racquetball pro can also match you up with other players. As for equipment costs, those are fairly modest. All you need is a decent racket, which can be had for less than $100 in sporting goods stores. Top-of-the-line rackets, however, will set you back more than $150.

Downhill Skiing

Skiing is a demanding physical activity that improves your strength, flexibility, and cardiovascular endurance, even more so because the sport is practiced at high altitude.

Skiing is one of those sports, however, that is better to get in shape *for* than to get in shape *from*. Those who ski while out of shape are susceptible to heart attacks. I've seen the ski patrol take away plenty of 50-year-old skiers (usually men) in their toboggans. It wasn't a pretty sight.

This winter sport has also become frighteningly expensive in the last ten years, but it's still an invigorating activity amongst the most beautiful outdoor scenery in the world.

Quick Hits

The following is a list of other sports or physical activities that we know from yesteryear, the contribution to an exercise or fitness program each provides, and the drawbacks:

- **Basketball**

    Premise: Running after loose balls, playing hard-nosed defense, and going to the hoop adds up to a heavy workout.

    Upside: Lots of short-spurt running and jumping. Easy to break a sweat.

    Downside: This is a guy's sport. Not many women 40 and up grew up playing basketball in the days before the passage of Title IX opened up athletic opportunities for high school and college females.

     The hardwood floor can be a killing field in terms of injuries.

- **Rowing (or crew)**

    Premise: Row, row, row your boat, a lot quicker than gently down the stream.

    Upside: Great strength-conditioning and aerobic exercise.

    Downside: Not too many people have learned to row, and it takes a lot of effort to take your scull to a nearby lake or river. If you row with others in two-person or four-person sculls, you have to organize your training sessions in advance.

- **Water skiing**

    Premise: Getting pulled by a speedboat results in an upper-body workout.

    Upside: Your arms and legs work hard to keep you upright and above water.

    Downside: You won't be able to comb your hair the next morning because your arms are so sore.

- **Volleyball**

    Premise: Lunging for balls and making kill shots provides a good workout.

    Upside: Lots of movement, quick digs for balls, and hustle.

    Downside: You have to be a skilled player and play in a top-end league to get the full fitness benefits of volleyball.

✔ **Hockey**

Premise: Slam-blam action on ice.

Upside: Terrific cardiovascular workout for those who can skate well.

Downside: Finding an old men's league and booking rink time, unless you like to play hockey from 1 to 3:30 a.m. (Hockey is also a guy's sport, for the same reasons as basketball.)

✔ **Soccer**

Premise: Slam-blam action on grass.

Upside: Terrific cardiovascular workout as you run up and down the field.

Downside: Must join a league; you can't play casually.

✔ **Softball**

Premise: Relive those glory days of Little League.

Upside: Everyone's a hitter in this slow-paced version of baseball.

Downside: You won't get into shape watching the grass grow in right field.

Chapter 21

Not Talking 'bout My Generation: New Fitness Activities

*I*n Chapter 20, I talk about familiar physical activities and appealing sports that we all like to play. Now I'm going to mix things up and discuss sporting pursuits that weren't even *invented* in our teenage and young adult years.

"But Betsy," you protest, "you can't teach an old dog new tricks."

Agreed, but you're never too old to stop learning. You know how to e-mail, right? (Oops, bad question.) Anyway, here are four sports and a hot aerobic activity that have popped up on the fitness radar screen in recent years. These athletic endeavors aren't difficult to master, with the exception of rock climbing. If you stay the course, however, these trendy sports can widen your fitness horizons while plastering your face with a satisfying ear-to-ear grin.

In-line Skating: Making the Right Moves

In-line skating, often incorrectly called rollerblading because a company called Rollerblade was one of the first to market in-line skates, has made huge strides in popularity. In less than 15 years, in-line skating came out of the blocks to become one of the top 20 participation sports in the United States.

Called the nation's fastest growing recreational activity, in-line skating is almost as simple as walking and appeals to a wide age group. Perhaps you've seen gray-haired grandmas whizzing by in the park or watched in awe as 20-year-old burrheads performed their loop-de-loops during ESPN's X-Games.

You don't have to skate in a half-pipe to enjoy this sport; in fact, I'd recommend against grinding rails and 360-degree midair grabs. Such shenanigans would likely pull every muscle in your body — and break a bone or two on the crash landing. But in-line skating through the park or on neighborhood sidewalks provides an excellent cardiovascular workout that targets key muscle groups. Although this low-impact sport requires a certain amount of strength in the knees for balance, in-line skating is easier on the joints than jogging or aerobic exercise. Skating naturally builds the hip and thigh muscles in ways that running and cycling do not. And you get an upper-arm workout when you swing your arms with each long stride.

The secrets of skating success

When you look at the benefits of in-line skating, you can easily see why this activity has grown so popular so quickly:

- ✔ **In-line skating is accessible.** You don't need a ballfield, ice rink, or swimming pool to participate — all you need is a ribbon of concrete. You can roll out of your driveway and cruise around the neighborhood or head to nearby parks and glide along uncrowded sidewalks (which many in-line skaters prefer).

- ✔ **In-line skating is inexpensive.** You can purchase a very good pair of recreational in-line skates for under $200; padding runs you another $75 to $100. Purchase recreational models for your skates, not the in-line hockey versions, because these skates are built for quick turns, which means less ankle support. You want four wheels, not three or five. Five wheels are harder to turn, and three wheels don't offer a stable ride; four wheels strike a balance between maneuverability and stability. After the initial cost of purchasing your skates, you don't have to worry about special facility costs, unless you're the adventurous sort and want to get your licks in at a skateboard park.

- ✔ **In-line skating is a great workout.** You reach your target heart rate in no time and gain all the benefits of regular exercise, including increased energy levels, lower blood pressure, and reduced risk of cancer and strokes. Studies have shown that in-line skating constitutes a more effective workout than cycling because cyclists glide more (and, therefore, work less).

Those who coast, toast their workout. Don't forget that the harder you skate, the more calories you burn; so remember to push off your skates to get your heartbeat up.

✔ **In-line skating is safe.** Serious injuries and death are rare occurrences in the sport; fewer than ten people die each year from in-line skating accidents. As a way of comparison, more than 800 bicyclists are killed annually. To skate safely, wearing a full set of gear — helmet, elbow and kneepads, and wrist guards — is mandatory. A recent study showed that 93 percent of injured skaters were *not* wearing full gear at the time of their accidents.

✔ **In-line skating is fun.** I've skated a few times, but I have to admit that I'm not very good at it. If I got any better, I can see where this fast, self-propelled sport would be a kick as you stroke and glide through the neighborhood.

✔ **In-line skating is a family sport.** Perhaps your children have been in-line skating since kindergarten and can skate circles around you. If so, great! From the elementary school years and up, you and the kids can embark on long rides together. Make sure your children have their helmets and pads on. No one wants to see someone you love break a bone or chip a tooth.

How to tell if in-line skating is for you

In-line skating is a good sport to try if

✔ **You ice skated as a young child.** Those who grew up playing hockey or ice skating on frozen ponds will make a smooth transition to in-line skating. Skating really is like riding a bike — your body doesn't forget.

✔ **You have good bike paths close to home.** In-line skaters need room to roam. Skating through parks is better than in neighborhoods, where you have to worry about dodging cars backing out of driveways or using little kids as human slalom poles.

✔ **You are looking for a low-impact alternative to jogging.** In-line skating is easier on the knees and ankles, placing 50 percent less impact on the joints than running. I must point out, though, that running works the heart and lungs better because in-line skaters glide from time to time.

✔ **You're looking for some adventure.** I admit that suiting up for in-line skating (donning the helmet, elbow and kneepads, and wrist guards) can be a bit daunting for neophytes. But if you're willing to give it a try, you may find that this is your sport.

Getting started; getting stopped

When you're learning how to in-line skate, recognize your limits and skate within them. Now is not the time to take on Suicide Hill. Develop your budding skating skills on level surfaces free from debris, fallen leaves, and cracks. Tennis courts and basketball courts are ideal. Make long strides and round turns, staying in control.

Ask a friend to teach you how to brake, which is a *very* important factor for avoiding emergency room visits. The ability to stop is crucial for in-line skaters. You'll enjoy yourself more when you aren't crashing into cars, pedestrians, fire hydrants, tiny tots, mailboxes, trees, bushes, baby carriages, and elderly walkers.

There are three main braking maneuvers:

- ✔ **The standard heel stop.** The brake is usually situated on the heel of the right skate. While rolling forward on both feet, keep your posture upright and knees relaxed. When you want to brake, stagger your right foot forward in a scissors-like move, lifting the right toe up until you feel the rubber brake rub against the concrete. Press the heel into the ground until you come to a stop. (*Note:* You won't be able to stop on a dime.)

- ✔ **The toe stop.** Some skates come equipped with a brake pad located on the toe of the skate. You stop by dragging the toe of the brake foot. Toe stops don't work very well on steep hills, though.

- ✔ **The dive.** You're striding along a sidewalk when a car suddenly pulls into the driveway. You have to stop *immediately*. Don't panic. Look for the nearest patch of grass and dive. Roll with the fall and then dust yourself off. Hopefully, the only injury is to your pride.

Gearing up

In-line skating without a helmet and pads is like playing hockey in a bathing suit. Sooner rather than later, you're going to fall and hit the deck. You escape road rash and serious injuries by donning protective gear.

- ✔ **Helmet.** Striking a curb, car, or concrete abutment with your head has serious medical and financial consequences. Bike helmets work fine; just be sure to wear one.

- ✔ **Knee and elbow guards.** These Darth Vader-like mixes of rugged black plastic, stretch fabric, and Velcro protect against injury to your joints. Experienced skaters use the kneepads to prevent injury by sliding on them during a fall; this dissipates energy and redistributes the force of striking the ground. Elbow pads protect the arms and elbows on sideways falls.

- ✔ **Wrist guards.** Wrist guards defend against the most common in-line skating injury: breaking or hyperextending the wrist when you try to break your fall with outstretched arms. Wrist guards offer protection against sprains, strains, and lacerations.

A close call

I'll never forget the first time I tried in-line skating. Iva Majoli, winner of the 1997 French Open, dropped by the house with some skates. Iva, who grew up in Croatia and probably started ice skating before she could ride a bike, skated circles around me in the driveway.

I tried on the pair of skates Iva had brought for me. I admit that I was a bit nervous as I put them on for the first time, along with the protective knee and elbow pads and wrist guards. I stood up and got going, but because I didn't know how to brake and like to go fast, I braked by jumping into the grass.

Then a few months later, I decided to take my then six-month-old daughter, Maggie, for a walk in one of those baby joggers (the type with three wheels). Except I wasn't walking; I had strapped on my in-line skates.

I'll spare you the details, but we nearly had a disaster when Maggie's cart started heading for the street — without me holding onto it. You should have seen me trying to grab the jogger while wearing those in-line skates. I managed to save the day, but not before gaining some appreciation for those who learned to skate at a young age.

Mountain Biking: Conquering More Than Hills

Perhaps you haven't noticed the fat-tire revolution in the world of cycling. Well, the war is over, and mountain bikes have won. In only 20 years, mountain bikes have supplanted the kinds of bikes we grew up with — three-speeds and ten-speeds — to become *the* most popular bike for the most popular cycling activity, mountain biking. Sales of mountain bikes outnumber all other bike sales combined, according to *Mountain Bike* magazine. More and more people are discovering that switching to dirt and outdoor scenery sure beats fighting traffic and pockmarked macadam.

Go hybrid

Not sure if you want the speed and power of a traditional road bike or the sturdiness and low gears of a mountain bike? Then split the difference!

This compromise between the two is called a hybrid bike, and it comes with upright handlebars so you can sit fairly straight, instead of in that hunched-over position you assume when you reach for a road bike's "dropped" handlebars. A wider seat, heavier frame, and wider tires handle dirt roads with assurance. The tires are not as wide as a mountain bike's, however, which means you go faster on asphalt. Plan on spending $400 to $1,000 for a decent hybrid.

The skinny on wide-tire biking

Mountain biking mirrors the exercise benefits found in skinny-tire cycling. You burn calories like a locomotive, strengthen the legs until they feel like anvils, and pump up your cardiovascular fitness to new heights. Mountain biking is a great way to combine physical activity with the Great Outdoors.

Mountain biking is easy to learn; everyone grew up riding a bike. Today's mountain bikes have 18 to 24 gears, easy-to-use controls, and wide, knobby tires that contribute to a stable ride. The robust suspension systems take out the bumpiness found on mountain-bike trails. Although mountain bikes are designed for off-road use, they also perform well on city streets. Some people prefer mountain biking on streets because the fat-tired bikes can easily negotiate sudden sections of sandy or pebble-strewn roadway.

When shopping for mountain bikes, let an independent bike retailer steer you in the right direction. You can pay up to $5,000, but you don't need to. Mountain bikes with great features, performance, and durability can be found for between $400 and $1,000.

Local bike shops are also repositories of information; look here for mountain bike clubs, organized group rides, maps of mountain bike trails close to home, and vacation hints.

Rules of the trail

The International Mountain Bicycling Association has come up with a list of rules for mountain bikers to follow:

- ✔ **Ride on open trails only.** Many cities have opened up areas for off-road cycling. Respect the trail signs. Don't trespass on private land; you wouldn't appreciate it if mountain bikers were riding on your property. If you live near a wilderness area, be aware that federal and state wilderness areas are closed to cycling.

- ✔ **Control your mountain bike.** Things happen quickly on the riding trail — chipmunks dart in front of you, boulders and small rocks appear out of nowhere, or erosion takes out part of the trail. Keep your speed under control so you can safely handle any of these contingencies.

- ✔ **Be ready to yield to hikers and other mountain bikers.** No walkers like to cringe while a mountain bike party scoots by, so announce your arrival ("Coming through") and slow down to a crawl as you pass pedestrians. Trails are often thin (called *single tracks*), so when other mountain bikes approach, slow way down so you can give each other plenty of room to get by. On other occasions, anticipate other trail users around bends or in blind spots.

- **Never spook animals, especially horses.** Take special care when passing horseback riders. Your sudden appearance can cause the horse to rear up and buck its rider off. Give the animals extra time to know that you're in the area. The same goes for hikers with dogs. Your patience gives the dog owner time to bring the animal under control and can save you from getting bitten. Finally, running cattle or disturbing other livestock is a serious offense; don't do it.

- **Plan ahead.** Planning ahead means having water and food with you when riding off-road, knowing your equipment and ability level, wearing a helmet, and carrying along supplies for changes in weather or other conditions.

- **Wear gloves and bike shorts.** You wouldn't think it, but gloves are an important accessory when mountain biking. Gloves absorb moisture, which gives you a better grip of the handlebars. Gloves come in handy if you happen to fall because you break falls by outstretching your arms. Gloves can also protect fingers from shrubs and prickly plants that droop over the trail. Bike shorts — those black Lycra jobs with padded gel liners — prevent leg chafing. Another chafe-prevention step is to wear bike shorts without undies.

And here's one of my rules for the road: If you're riding on a mountain bike trail, be environmentally friendly by keeping your fat tires in the middle of the trail. If you fail to steer precisely, you widen the trail, and we all know that taking the trail less traveled is good for nature and good for us.

Gear talk

If you're going to start mountain biking, pocket some of these slang words to impress your friends:

- **Babyheads:** Roundish rocks found in loose jumbles on hairpin corners.

- **Bacon:** Scabs on rider's knees, elbows, or other body parts.

- **Chunder:** To crash.

- **Endo:** Flying unexpectedly over the handlebars.

- **Lid:** Helmet. Also known as a "skid lid."

- **Fred:** Someone who spends much money on a mountain bike but still can't ride; for example, "What a fred — too much Lycra and titanium." Also known as a "barney" or "poser."

- **POD:** A Potential Organ Donor; bad rider.

- **Potato chip:** A badly bent wheel; a wheel that is bent completely over is considered "taco-ed."

- **Yard sale:** A horrendous crash that strews your wares — water bottle, pump, tool bag, and bike — all over the trail.

Snowboarding: Let's Carve, Dude!

Dave and Stephanie Nelson — friends call her Stevie — have been living in Mammoth Lakes, California, home of Mammoth Mountain, since their ski-bum days back in the 1970s. Perhaps you've never heard of Mammoth, but this Alpine-like resort high in the Eastern Sierra Nevada mountain range is one of the nation's busiest ski areas, thanks to its proximity to Los Angeles skiers.

Dave and Stevie became managers of a large condominium complex in Mammoth, settled down, and began raising a family. The proud parents put Natalie and Chris Nelson on skis not long after they learned to walk, but when their kids' friends took up a new sport called snowboarding in the late 1980s, Natalie and Chris had to try "boarding" as well. Natalie and Chris ditched their skis and began slashing Mammoth's slopes with their snowboards; when they reached their teens, the kids were competing in national snowboarding events.

At first, Dave and Stevie thought snowboarding was too dangerous and attracted a wild crowd. As this alternative sport matured and outgrew its outlaw image, however, Dave and Stevie — die-hard skiers in their early forties — decided to give snowboarding a try.

They loved it! Dave and Stevie sold their old skis and began snowboarding several times a week. What they've also found is that as they have gotten older, snowboarding has been a great way to restore old friendships and have fun with friends their age. "Stevie and I like having friends to board with," said Dave. "Sometimes the guys will go one direction and the gals will go another, and we'll meet up for lunch. Snowboarding is a fun couples activity that builds relationships. It's like doing something new together."

Hitting the slopes (literally)

Dave and Stevie say that you're never too old to start snowboarding. Just keep in mind the following points:

- **Snowboarding has a steep learning curve.** If you expect to strap on a board and ride down the ski trail right away, you have another thing coming. First-time snowboarders become frustrated from continually falling and pushing themselves up again. Unless you're a gifted athlete or grew up surfing, several days will pass before you start to feel comfortable riding a snowboard. You can't commit only one day to learning this sport. Commit three days. The first day you feel foolish; the second day you get the hang of it; and the third day you're off and boarding. If you can, start snowboarding with your spouse or a good friend — overcoming beginner's embarrassment is easier with someone you know.

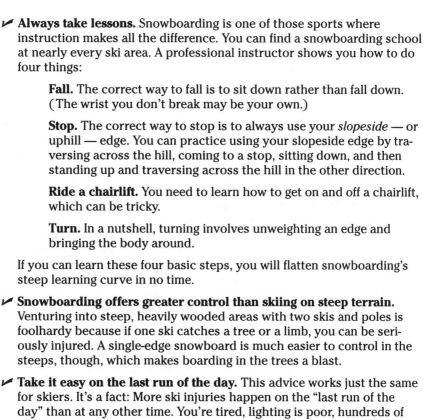

✔ **Always take lessons.** Snowboarding is one of those sports where instruction makes all the difference. You can find a snowboarding school at nearly every ski area. A professional instructor shows you how to do four things:

> **Fall.** The correct way to fall is to sit down rather than fall down. (The wrist you don't break may be your own.)

> **Stop.** The correct way to stop is to always use your *slopeside* — or uphill — edge. You can practice using your slopeside edge by traversing across the hill, coming to a stop, sitting down, and then standing up and traversing across the hill in the other direction.

> **Ride a chairlift.** You need to learn how to get on and off a chairlift, which can be tricky.

> **Turn.** In a nutshell, turning involves unweighting an edge and bringing the body around.

If you can learn these four basic steps, you will flatten snowboarding's steep learning curve in no time.

✔ **Snowboarding offers greater control than skiing on steep terrain.** Venturing into steep, heavily wooded areas with two skis and poles is foolhardy because if one ski catches a tree or a limb, you can be seriously injured. A single-edge snowboard is much easier to control in the steeps, though, which makes boarding in the trees a blast.

✔ **Take it easy on the last run of the day.** This advice works just the same for skiers. It's a fact: More ski injuries happen on the "last run of the day" than at any other time. You're tired, lighting is poor, hundreds of skiers are descending the mountain simultaneously, and there's the temptation to just let it go and bomb down the hill. Those are all ingredients for a major crash and a one-way trip in the ski patrol toboggan.

The benefits of boarding

In less than 30 years, snowboarding has become a mainstream sport. The sport started with an outlaw image as hell-bent-for-leather snowboarders — mainly young males ages 14 to 24 — took over the mountain, but those days are past. Men and women of all ages and sizes are learning how to snowboard down the mountain for the following reasons:

✔ **Snowboarding increases muscular strength, flexibility, and overall fitness.** You're going to be sore after snowboarding because you're using muscles you thought you never had and because you're pushing yourself off the snow all day long. Believe me, the Jacuzzi will never look better than after your first day on the slopes. As you get better and don't fall so much, you find that snowboarding works your calves, gluteus muscles, hamstrings, and quadriceps.

✔ **Snowboarding is easier on your knees than downhill skiing.** Dave Nelson says he's taught many friends to snowboard, including Ed McGlasson, a retired 300-pound NFL center now in his forties. Pro football destroyed Ed's knees, but he gave snowboarding a shot with Dave's help. Ed, who had to wear braces when he snow skied, was amazed that he could snowboard without pain and that his knees were "just fine."

✔ **Your lungs get exercised from having to suck in all that rarefied air.** Snowboarding takes place in altitude, meaning that the smaller amount of oxygen in the air forces your lungs and heart to work harder.

Equipping yourself for the ride

Snowboarding kicked around the fringes of winter sports in the 1970s as various inventors experimented with bolting skis together, sliding down the hill on cafeteria trays, and transforming surfboards into "wintersticks." As each new generation of snowboards advanced the sport, the media began picking up on "snurfers" who rode on the snow much like a surfer carved turns on the face of a wave. By the mid-1980s, snowboarding caught on with young, thrill-seeking males, and a new winter ski experience was born.

It probably won't be too long before snowboarders outnumber skiers. If you're willing to ski out of your comfort zone, then consider trying to snowboard on your next winter trip.

Modern snowboards come in three types:

✔ **Freestyle:** A board made for performing tricks and suitable for beginners.

✔ **Freeriding:** An all-purpose board also suitable for beginners.

✔ **Carving:** A board designed for high-speed, giant slalom-like turns.

Unless you ski more than two weeks a year, you should rent. You can try other boards in different lengths, weight, and styles. Rent soft boots as well, although you may consider purchasing snowboarding boots, which could have other uses like walking around the ski resort or trudging through heavy snow at home. Leave the hard-shelled boots for snowboard racers.

Wear shell parkas and baggy pants that don't restrict movement. Wear several layers of clothes underneath to stay warm. Insulated, waterproof pants usually come with built-in padded knees, which come in handy for kneeling in the snow during your day on the slopes.

Don't chintz on gloves. Snowboarders put their hands on the snow a lot, so buy extra-long, Gore-Tex-like gloves that keep the fingers and hands warm.

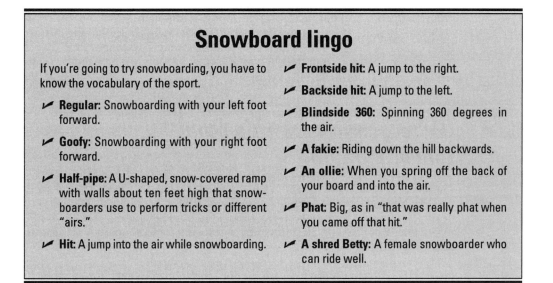

Snowboard lingo

If you're going to try snowboarding, you have to know the vocabulary of the sport.

- **Regular:** Snowboarding with your left foot forward.

- **Goofy:** Snowboarding with your right foot forward.

- **Half-pipe:** A U-shaped, snow-covered ramp with walls about ten feet high that snowboarders use to perform tricks or different "airs."

- **Hit:** A jump into the air while snowboarding.

- **Frontside hit:** A jump to the right.

- **Backside hit:** A jump to the left.

- **Blindside 360:** Spinning 360 degrees in the air.

- **A fakie:** Riding down the hill backwards.

- **An ollie:** When you spring off the back of your board and into the air.

- **Phat:** Big, as in "that was really phat when you came off that hit."

- **A shred Betty:** A female snowboarder who can ride well.

Rock Climbing: Going Up?

Word association time.

When I say "rock climbing," what words pop into your mind?

Extreme sport.

Daredevil activity.

Shortened life span.

I would have to agree. Scaling sheer walls, towering spires, and mountain summits tethered to a rope and hanging hundreds if not thousands of feet above *terra firma* certainly sounds like a dangerous sport to me.

Yet for all its danger, rock climbing has become mainstream and has doubled its national participants in the last ten years; the American Sports Climbers Federation counts 1 million rock climbing enthusiasts today.

I can't say that rock climbing holds much interest for me — I haven't climbed anything higher than the Bakers' tree fort when I was in sixth grade. I will not dispute, however, that this unique form of taxing exercise uses every muscle group in the body — not just the upper body — and increases hand-eye coordination, balance, strength, and flexibility. Interestingly, rock climbing is a great equalizer between the sexes because the strength-to-weight ratio makes it easier for women to pull themselves up, especially on negative-incline walls found at most indoor climbing gyms.

We're gonna rock this gym: Indoor climbing

The sport of rock climbing forces participants to face their fears: fear of heights, fear of falling, and fear of equipment failure. I could add "fear of death," but I don't want to talk about *that* kind of rock climbing (the kind where you try to imitate Spiderman by inching up 5.14d sandstone walls outside Moab, Utah).

Instead, I want to shift the focus to indoor "rock gyms," where you're more likely to see participants from your age group. The inherent risks of indoor climbing are manageable because of the controlled environment. (And it does help that you're never more than 30 feet off the ground.)

If you're thinking about giving indoor rock climbing a try, you won't be allowed to scale an artificial wall without taking an introductory course, which usually lasts for three hours and is often free. An introductory lesson covers

✔ Safety rules.

✔ How to tie yourself into a harness.

✔ Various holds and climbing maneuvers.

✔ How to tie basic mountaineering knots, such as the figure-eights.

✔ How to belay.

Belaying is one of the essential aspects of rock climbing. To *belay* means to stand on the ground and hold the safety rope while your partner ascends the wall. The belayer is responsible for taking up the slack of the rope so the climber falls just a few inches in case he or she loses a grip or foothold. (Be careful when you're on the ground. You can get "belayer's neck" from constantly looking upward. Try to rotate belaying duties with others.)

Fortunately, falls are fairly rare in indoor climbing. Rock climbers are more likely to develop tendonitis in their fingers and wrists because of the great strains placed on these muscles and ligaments while climbing.

What you can expect to pay

Equipment costs are about the same as in-line skating: $300. You need to purchase rock shoes — lightweight shoes with tough soles that help you grab, hold, and interact with the rock and touch points on the artificial wall. You also need a set of *carabiners* — metal snapping links used in various climbing tasks — climbing rope, and a harness that fits snugly but not too tightly.

Indoor rock climbing gyms sell full-day passes for $10 to $30, depending on the metropolitan area. Monthly dues are more reasonable. You can learn more about the sport by contacting your local indoor climbing center. Rock climbing is not a skill learned in two afternoon introductory sessions, however. You can expect to spend months acquiring the ability to scale indoor walls from bottom to top.

Tae-Bo: It's New and It's Hot

In the beginning, God created fitness centers and said, "Let there be aerobics." And all across the grassy plain, aerobics classes multiplied and were fruitful.

But the people became bored and demanded more, so God created step aerobics. Again, step aerobics multiplied and was fruitful, but the people became bored.

So God raised up a man named Billy Blanks to lead his people out of the fitness wilderness. Billy stepped forth and introduced a feverish, nonstop routine of high steps, kicks, and punches called *Tae-Bo*. The people followed Billy in droves, and fitness came across the land.

Thanks for letting me have some fun with Tae-Bo, the latest fitness fad. Set to energetic hip-hop music, this form of cardio-kickboxing combines the intensity and high enthusiasm of aerobic dance with the self-defense moves of martial arts. Billy Blanks, who invented Tae-Bo, has amassed a fortune since his first infomercial aired in August 1998.

There's no doubt that Tae-Bo delivers a whole body workout that tones and defines muscles, improves balance and coordination, and combines low impact and high-intensity aerobic exercise. Tae-Bo burns calories by the bushelful, too — around 350 to 450 per hour for a 135-pound woman, according to a University of Mississippi study. You also work up a flop sweat, if you mimic Billy and his students as they kick and punch the air on the instructional tapes.

To go where no man has gone before

We haven't reached the final recreational frontier yet — not by a long shot or a short toss. We are sure to see new sports, new fitness regimens, and new variations of old sports in coming years. As long as there's money and an infomercial to be made, entrepreneurs will attempt to build a better fitness mousetrap.

Balf

A new sport that's a hybrid of baseball and golf — called *balf* — is being kicked around by its inventor Mark Schuster of Crafton, Pennsylvania. (Balf, which rhymes with *golf*, comes from a combination of BAseball and goLF.) Billing itself "The Sport of the Third Millennium," balf is played on golf courses using golf balls and special wooden bats known as "clats."

The player stands on the tee box, tosses the golf ball into the air, and swings from the heels. Call it fungo golf. Hopefully, the ball lands in the fairway, where the player picks up the ball again and smacks it toward the hole. Once on the green, the player uses a special clat with a putter head to putt the ball into the hole. You can become a charter member of the U.S. Balf Association (or learn more about this fledgling game) by going online at www.balf.com.

Snag

Another golf-like game to watch for is called Snag, which is a form of "soft golf" that can be played in cul-de-sacs and parks — anywhere you can hit 100-yard shots. Players hit a Velcro-like tennis ball with a specially made club toward a "flagstickie." Former PGA touring pro Wally Armstrong, a fellow Orlando resident, is bringing this new game to market.

Goaltimate

If you liked tossing a Frisbee as a kid, you should try Goaltimate, a game played by two teams trying to throw a flying disc (such as a Frisbee) through an 11-foot arch. Players run a lot, trying to intercept Frisbee passes, and the game has taken hold in Boston and San Diego. "With Goaltimate, it's like running a marathon," says Rick Conner, a San Diegan who's trying to take the sport into the mainstream. "There's no downtime." You can find out more by going to www.goaltimate.com.

Kiteboarding

Water and wind enthusiasts may want to check out kiteboarding, a cross between windsurfing and parasailing. Strapping themselves on windsurfing boards, thrill-seekers launch a XXL-sized kite into the wind and take off — sometimes literally. Kiteboaders have been known to land in trees or parking lots when a sudden gust of wind lifted them and their boards into the heavens. (These adrenaline-rush moments are called "kitemares" by participants.)

Not for the faint of heart, kiteboarding has gained a foothold in the trade winds of Maui, where several kiteboarding schools have opened up in recent years. For more information about this new sport, Web surf at www.kitehigh.com.

Tae-Bo is not for fitness beginners. Many exercises involve standing on one leg and kicking parallel to the floor, which can put you at risk for hip, knee, and low-back injuries. If you decide to try Tae-Bo, start slowly and work your way up the fitness ladder.

There are only two ways you can do Tae-Bo: (1) by purchasing Billy's four-video series (around $60) and following along at home, or (2) by flying to the Billy Blanks World Training Center in Los Angeles' San Fernando Valley, where Billy and his handpicked trainers put classes through their paces. (Sinbad, Carmen Electra, Brooke Shields, and Paula Abdul have dropped by to kick and shout.) Women seem to be drawn to Tae-Bo more than men, which mirrors the male/female participation rates in aerobics and step aerobics classes.

Vita parcours

They seem so retro, so '60s, so out of place if you happen to stumble across one these days. They're called *parcours*, and they were introduced in our teenage years. Finding one in decent shape is hard to do these days. Many are rusting away like old VW campers parked outside a Grateful Dead concert.

You may be caught in a time warp, wondering *parcours . . . parcours . . . I know I've heard that word before.* Let me offer a snap refresher course. A parcours is a running course with exercise stations. Back in the mid-1960s, a Swiss architect named Erwin Weckemann had a brainstorm: design an exercise course with 20 or more wood-and-metal exercise stations scattered at intervals along a dirt jogging trail. People could jog from station to station, pausing long enough to carry out each of the 20 exercises (chin-ups, sideway jumps, push-ups, calf raises, and so on). Herr Weckemann prevailed upon Vita, a Zurich-based life insurance company, to sponsor the construction of the world's first *parcours.*

Each station carried a sign with exercise instructions. The system seemed to combine play and exercise and fresh air, which appealed to the Swiss. By the early 1970s, Switzerland boasted more than 200 *parcours,* and the idea soon spread through Western Europe and the U.S. The first *parcours* was erected in the United States in 1973 at San Francisco's Mountain Lake Park. Hand-routed wooden signs guided the way. Then Perrier, the French mineral water bottler seeking to brand itself in the States, sponsored more than 200 parcours in major cities.

Parcours was anglicized to parcourse, and during the fitness boom of the 1980s, close to 4,500 were built from sea to shining sea. Parks, riverbeds, industrial parks, bike paths — almost anywhere with room for a mile-long circular trail of exercise stations — became home to a parcourse. Then, just like that, parcourses fell into disuse as sales of home exercise equipment sharply rose in the late 1980s and 1990s and low-cost fitness gyms began popping up in mini-malls. The parcourse demise is too bad because the exercise stations lead you through a step-by-step, balanced, full-body workout in around 30 to 45 minutes, with plenty of stretching, limbering, strengthening, and cardiovascular workouts. There's something refreshingly low-tech about exercising at free, outdoor calisthenics stations, gulping fresh air by the lungful as you perform a new exercise every few minutes.

I don't know what the future holds for parcourses. My guess is that they will end up on the trash heap of fitnessdom. Parcourses, an antidote to the mind-numbing monotony of treadmills and steppers, deserve a better fate. If you happen to visit your local parcourse after years of being away, don't be surprised if you're alone — unless you count the ants and beetles chewing away on the rotting wood platforms.

Like any fitness program, do Tae-Bo at least three times a week for maximum benefit. While I've heard that Tae-Bo can be fun, I can't see how playing the same Tae-Bo videos over and over can keep anyone's interest level high for the long run. If nothing else, use Tae-Bo as a change-of-pace, moderate-impact aerobic activity that's part of a varied fitness routine.

You do have one other avenue for Tae-Bo-like exercise: You may see advertisements for kickboxing aerobics at your local fitness gym. These copycat programs cannot call themselves "Tae-Bo" workouts (that word is trademarked by Billy Blanks), but they may be worth checking out.

Chapter 22

Unique Ways to Work Out

. . . .

In This Chapter

▶ Chilling out with yoga and tai chi: mind-body exercises

▶ Jumping on the Pilates bandwagon

▶ Using magnets

▶ Home cookin': low-tech ways to work out in your living room or patio area

. . . .

A big part of staying fit over 40 is determination — keeping that appointment with yourself to exercise. Only *you* can drag yourself out of bed for that early morning walk or aerobics class at the gym. Only *you* can stop your workday for a noontime stint in the corporate fitness room. Only *you* can squeeze in exercise between work and dinner.

The discipline involved in bringing fitness to the forefront and making lifestyle changes is not easy to wrangle; you must put your mind to it. In a sense, committing to a fitness regimen is like putting mind over matter, except in this case, your body is the matter!

Which leads me to this chapter about "mind-body" exercises (such as yoga and tai chi) and overlooked exercises you can do at home — if you put your mind to it. Each discipline can be a route to physical nirvana, which is why these sure-fire health enhancers deserve a look. If you wrestle with staying motivated about fitness, perhaps these different routes to fitness will keep you focused on the goal — being fit after 40.

Doing Mind-Body Exercises: Where Spiritual and Physical Meet

Yoga, tai chi, and Pilates are called "mind-body" exercises because the mind and body work together toward a common goal. These three disciplines show you how to get in touch with your body, which, when you stop to think about it, cannot be disassociated from the mind. I believe that when you change the body on a physical level, you also change it on the mental level — a mind-body connection.

Let me explain further. The mind-body connection is the mechanism that drives all the voluntary and involuntary actions of the body, and it's hard to separate the two. I know that my physical activities and continuous exercise have influenced my mental outlook over the years, and my mental outlook exerts a powerful influence on the way I feel physically and spiritually. I always play better tennis matches — perform well athletically — when my mind is calm, uncluttered, and alert. The same principle is the foundation of yoga, tai chi, and Pilates. These disciplines not only take inches off your thighs and mid-section, but they can reduce everyday stress and give you the confidence you need to operate at a "higher level of consciousness," as their proponents claim.

I admit up front, however, that I am out of my league when it comes to mind-body exercises such as yoga or tai chi, mainly because I feel these exercise forms reveal more about one's worldview regarding spiritual matters than about a desire to become physically fit. Taking a yoga or tai chi class is fine, and the choreographed patterns of movements, called *forms*, improve cardio-vascular endurance, posture, strength, and balance. But make no mistake about it: You can't separate the spiritual from the physical when it comes to yoga and tai chi, and, to a lesser extent, Pilates. Here's what I mean:

- ✔ **Yoga** places an emphasis on breathing and meditation, but this spiritual discipline from India, partly based on Hinduism, essentially seeks to liberate the individual from the illusory world of phenomena and achieve a state called *samadhi*, or dissolution of the personality. Translation: Yoga isn't merely physical. When you create outer strength, you also create inner strength. Yoga practitioners blend physical aspects of yoga (called *hatha yoga*) with forms of spiritual meditation. Some yoga classes emphasize the spiritual aspect, while others secularize it.

- ✔ **Tai chi** is an ancient martial art based on Taoist philosophy, which has adopted many features from Buddhism. The *tao*, in the broadest sense, is the way the universe functions, the path (the Chinese word *tao* means "path") taken by natural events. Man, following the *tao*, must give up all striving. His ideal state of being, fully attainable by mystical contemplation alone through meditation, is freedom from desire and from sensory experience, which is viewed as an illusion. Translation: The path to all-around being is through the practice of tai chi movements and meditation.

- ✔ **Pilates** (pronounced *pi-lah-teez*), a series of low-impact flexibility and muscle exercises, was developed by a German fitness guru named Joseph Pilates back in the 1920s. Pilates introduced a concept called Contrology in a book of exercises called *Return to Life Through Contrology*, in which he stated, "Contrology is complete coordination of body, mind, and spirit. Through Contrology, you first purposely acquire complete control of your own body, and then through proper repetition of its exercises, you gradually and progressively acquire that natural rhythm and coordination associated with all your subconscious activities." Translation: Pilates exercises put you in great physical shape and improve your mental outlook.

Practicing yoga and tai chi

I have no doubt that yoga and tai chi have fitness benefits. On my trips to China, I've seen the Chinese people, young and old alike, practice tai chi in public parks, making slow, graceful, ballet-like movements. They believe that the continuously changing series of postures achieves a harmonious flow of energy throughout the body. Tai chi has a slow-motion, dance-like quality that hides its true combat origins. Through the gradual building of one's inner energy, known as *chi,* one discovers how soft truly does overcome hard and how, in combat, an ounce of energy can defeat a thousand pounds of force.

Well, that's the thinking anyway. If you decide to take a class in yoga or tai chi, concentrate on the physical movements and realize that the spiritual underpinnings have nothing to do with fitness; but that's my opinion.

I want to put a good word in for deep-breathing exercises, which are great benefits of yoga and tai chi. When I play tennis, coaches harp on the importance of taking deep breaths during changeovers. Deep breathing certainly helps calm me down so I can think about the next game.

I have found this form of exercise highly beneficial in my work as a television commentator for ESPN. In the last five or ten minutes until we "go live," I become very nervous — more nervous than I ever was on Wimbledon's Centre Court. The thought of speaking eruditely while keeping my poise causes me to shiver in my sneakers. I have told the producer just before airtime that I need to take a time-out and do some deep-breathing exercises. Deep breathing is not a cure-all for stage fright, but I know I've been much calmer and collected after having slowed my body down.

Pulling for Pilates: No longer a well-kept secret

A mind-body fitness activity that looks promising is Pilates. I admit that I had not heard of Pilates until a couple of years ago, but the mainstream media has discovered this low-impact exercise program that promotes control of the mind, body, and spirit. Pilates was developed more than 70 years ago by Joseph Pilates, a German immigrant. The exercise regimen gained a foothold in New York City among the choreographers and dancers on Broadway. Today, Pilates has a bandwagon of interest, and it doesn't hurt that A-list celebrities such as Jamie Lee Curtis, Madonna, and Danny Glover have jumped aboard.

To do Pilates, you have to go to a Pilates studio, where an instructor leads you through a series of exercises or mat work. Most start from a supine position and involve lifting and strengthening some combination of arms, legs, and back. A heavier workout occurs when you subject yourself to special Pilates equipment that works your muscles with springs and pulleys. The machines stretch and elongate the muscles and joints, but Pilates instructors say that all movements must be generated from the *powerhouse*, or the central body muscles in the abdomen that connect to your lower back and buttocks. After you build up your stomach muscles, you can work on other parts of the body.

As for the mind-body aspect, Pilates was described as a "mix of yoga and Jane Fonda, with a dash of tai chi thrown in" by a *Newsweek* reporter. I'll have to take her word because I haven't experienced Pilates firsthand. But I have heard good results from friends and acquaintances, including a 45-year-old tennis player with a bad back for more than a year. She tried physical therapy and chiropractors without success, but when a friend suggested Pilates, the intense hour-long workouts strengthened her back and allowed her to resume playing tennis. "I came out of the studio dripping," she said. "What a workout!" She eventually had to stop her Pilates appointments because they are expensive (you pay $35 to $75 an hour).

Using a Magnetic Pull

Mike Yorkey, who's assisting me with this manuscript, attended a senior pro tennis tournament not long ago in San Diego. The tournament site was filled with product booths, and Mike visited a producer of magnetic bracelets designed to be worn around the wrists. He had read a *Golf Digest* story about the senior tour players who slept on beds of magnets or slapped magnetic bracelets on their right wrists — and experienced immediate pain relief for various aches and pains. The article stated that close to 90 percent of the senior players use magnets.

Mike's right wrist had been bothering him for several years because he sits in front of a computer and types all day. A hand surgeon told him that he didn't have carpal tunnel syndrome, but he probably suffered from some form of tendonitis. The surgeon counseled Mike to ride an exercise bike three times a week and get his heart rate way up, which would pump more blood through-out the body, including the right wrist. Exercise helped, but his right wrist was still so sore that he trained himself to use his mouse with his left hand.

Mike eyeballed the magnetic bracelets at the tennis booth. "Do these really work?" he asked.

Of course he was told, "Yes," but then the company representative said some-thing interesting: "They work even if you don't believe they'll work." *Yeah, right,* Mike thought. But he decided to give a magnetic bracelet a try — and his wrist stopping hurting!

Why do magnets supposedly work? It has something to do with increasing circulation in the body — a form of acupuncture. Remember how the hand surgeon told Mike that increased circulation could help his wrist pain? Same idea.

I received mixed results the one time I tried "magnetic therapy." I was in Hawaii with a sore knee and tennis elbow. A woman I met said she could help me find relief by having me hold two magnetic balls next to my bum knee and sore elbow. The knee didn't improve — and I'm not sure magnets could have helped my bone problem — but my elbow did feel better.

Employing Exercise Videos

Let's turn our attention to overlooked exercises that you can do at home — if you put your mind to it. A popular exercise option these days is to pop a video into the VCR and perform stretches and aerobic exercises in tune with the chirpy leader on screen. I have mixed reactions to exercise videos: Some are very good at what they do (giving you a complete workout), while others are campy efforts that have been around so long that they are ripe for parody. Personally, I've preferred to go outside and exercise, but that's easy to do in Florida's year-round climate.

Deciding whether videos are right for you

Although fitness videos can be exercises in cheesiness, and it's easy to poke fun at the cloying hosts and annoying antics, they do have their place in the pantheon of fitness. Exercise videos may work for you if you can answer yes to these questions:

✔ Do you live far from a health club? Many people live in rural areas or in city outskirts that are too far from a fitness facility.

✔ Are you housebound? Perhaps you are taking care of an aging parent or special needs child and can't leave the home.

✔ Do you live in a cold-weather climate that makes it difficult to leave the house during the winter?

✔ Do you have a limited budget? If you can't afford to purchase home fitness equipment, exercise videos are a stopgap measure.

✔ Is your space limited where home-exercise equipment is concerned? We don't all live in homes with extra room for a treadmill or exercise bike.

✔ Do you prefer the privacy of your home? Some folks don't want to exercise with others.

✔ Do you realize the limitations of exercise videos? You're alone with just an exercise mat and perhaps a couple of dumbbells and a kitchen "step" piece. You'll probably get a nice cardiovascular workout, but don't expect to do much strength training unless you use a video that includes dumbbells.

If you think you and exercise videos would be a good match, ask friends for recommendations. Personal trainers can point you in the right direction. Research the Internet. You'll always find a new someone who's "hot."

Most "active videos" cost between $15 and $20 and last for 45 minutes. I would not recommend purchasing exercise videos because they become boring after the fifth or sixth viewing and can actually become a "demotivator." A better route would be to ask friends if you can borrow their exercise videos or drop by your public library or video store, which should be stocked with dozens of fitness titles. Garage sales are another place where you'll find old fitness videos for pennies on the dollar.

Choosing the right tape

You'll find *hundreds* of exercise videos out there, all vying for a place in your VCR. Videos based on yoga, martial arts, jumping rope, kickboxing, aerobics, step aerobics, and stretching are everywhere. Rent or borrow an exercise video that you would never purchase. Experiment!

Before buying, renting, or borrowing an exercise video, however, you need to know whom the intended audience is supposed to be. Are you on the fitness comeback trail and need a video filled with slow stretches and easy movements? Or would you prefer something more energetic? Of course, you want a video where proper form is demonstrated and explained, so you won't injure yourself when performing the exercises.

Read the verbiage on the video jacket. "Low impact" means that one foot is always in contact with the floor. "High impact" indicates that both feet leave the floor during jumping or hopping moves. "Mixed impact" refers to a combination of both low-impact and high-impact moves during the aerobic portion or the addition of jump moves during step aerobics.

What does the video jacket say about intensity of the workout? Search for clues that reveal how difficult the workout is in relation to exercise selection, sequence, and complexity. Look for the following words on the video jacket verbiage:

- ✔ **Beginner** means you haven't exercised for a half year or longer. Your aerobic capacity, strength, and flexibility are suspect. You aren't sure how to monitor your heart rate to determine how much you are exercising.

- ✔ **Intermediate** means you're back on track, exercising consistently at least twice a week. You are familiar with the importance of stretching and are versed in various types of aerobic activities.

- ✔ **Advanced** means that you are in excellent shape, exercise three to five times a week, and can follow more complex routines. You know all about dance aerobics, step aerobics, and other modes of body conditioning. You feel fit and trim and have good coordination around the exercise floor.

Using the Venerable Jump Rope

Perhaps you haven't jumped rope since your best friends in third grade twirled a clothesline while you hopped in pigtails. Not to worry. The decidedly low-tech jump rope is still an effective way to burn fat, increase stamina, firm up muscles, improve coordination, and get exercise in a hurry. When I was playing on the pro tennis tour, I always kept a jump rope in my racket bag because I knew that jumping rope could be done anywhere at any time. I jumped in hotel rooms, in locker rooms, and courtside for years.

If you jumped rope as a youngster, you haven't forgotten how it's done. I admit that this form of exercise feels 20 times harder in your forties and fifties than it did in your grammar school days, when you never got winded. If you didn't jump rope as a youngster, however, jumping rope now takes some practice. You may get frustrated making two or three jumps and flubbing up. Hang in there and keep trying!

You need to stick with it because five minutes of jumping rope goes a long way in your adult years. This simple exercise is easier on your knees and ankles than running. If you work your way up to 15 minutes of moderate speed rope-jumping, you burn between 150 and 200 calories. But that level takes some time to reach because this intense, load-bearing exercise quickly works the lower legs. Don't be surprised if you run out of gas after a few minutes of skipping rope.

The old jump rope has lots going for it. It's cheap ($5 to $15), portable, and easy to use. Business travelers can use jump ropes in their hotel rooms (if the ceiling is high enough) or in the courtyard. Be sure to purchase one made of plastic or plastic beads with swivel handles. Leather jump ropes apparently take time to break in. Jump ropes come in different lengths, so ask a salesperson to fit you. A perfect fit occurs when you stand on the center of the rope with one foot and pull the rope straight up along both sides of your body. If the handles reach to your armpits, you're ready to begin. So start jumping like a jack!

Chapter 23

Massage: A Healthy Indulgence

Staying fit is twice as hard after 40 as it was when we were at our physical peaks in our late teens and early twenties. Mid-life fitness requires iron discipline, rock-hard determination, and extraordinary effort.

Fortunately, we usually have higher incomes at this stage of our lives. Our careers are in full bloom, which means our earning power is higher than it's ever been. If we've pushed the kids through college and are reaping the benefits of an empty nest, we may have a few extra bucks jangling in our pockets — unless that prestigious university our children attended swept up all our savings.

I can think of few better places to spend mad money than on a massage. Yes, a massage is a luxury item, but if you're going to indulge, here's the place to let yourself go. I speak from experience; my body has been the beneficiary of the work performed by skilled massage therapists since the early days of my professional tennis career.

Massage, bodywork, therapeutic massage — whatever you call it — is a worthy treat, but it also has physiological benefits. It will get your blood flowing, soothe jagged nerves, reduce adhesions in muscles and connective tissues, purge the body of wastes, speed up the removal of toxins, and make you feel *awesome*. The most common explanation for these health benefits is that massage therapy improves blood circulation, which enhances the body's capability to flush lactic acid build-up in the muscles. The fact that you feel refreshed and vitalized by a massage is testament to the power of the healing touch.

BETSY'S RACKET

An old profession — but not the oldest

The art of massage dates back to when the ancient Greeks carried around bottles of scented oil for their daily rubs. Twenty-five hundred years later, the demand for massage therapy has exploded here in the United States, thanks to the growing population of tired, aging, no-longer-limber baby boomers, who have the incomes and inclination to take advantage of the physiological benefits of pressing the flesh. Consumers visit massage therapists more than 114 million times per year, according to the *Journal of the American Medical Association,* and 41 percent of those massages are on bodies in the 45- to 64-year-old age bracket.

Since retiring from the professional tennis tour, I've been fortunate to be able to afford a massage therapist, and my twice-monthly massages with licensed therapist Steven Mercer are an indulgence that's better than pigging out with my favorite dessert: Häagen-Dazs Vanilla Swiss Almond ice cream topped with chocolate sauce. Steven is a much-in-demand massage therapist who's big with pro golfers based in Orlando, such as Mark O'Meara, Stuart Appleby, and some guy named Tiger.

Steven doesn't like to say that he gives "massages." He prefers a more honorable term known as "bodywork." I don't blame him. Massage has a seedy reputation in many parts of the world because some people can't say the word "massage" without linking it with the word "parlor." We all know that some massage parlors are just a front for prostitution. Steven and his cohorts do great work that's nothing close to seedy. As the advertisement used to say, "Try it, you'll like it."

But you knew that, right? Even if you have never employed the services of a professional massage therapist, you've probably enjoyed having your muscles tenderized by loved ones over the years. A back rub never goes out of style, and I've trained my husband, Mark, in the fine art of the back rub. Mark has been an excellent student; today, he's very good at giving back rubs. I just need to get him to stay with it longer than ten minutes.

Understanding the Different Types of Massage

A professional massage is more than a glorified back rub. If you're new to massage therapy, be aware of what kind of massage you're going to receive. Massage therapists can offer many variations on the massage theme. These are the main categories:

✔ **Swedish massage:** I'm sorry to be the one to tell you this, but you will not be worked over by a blond Nordic god or goddess with a golden touch after signing up for a Swedish massage. A Swedish massage happens when the therapist applies oil to your skin and then uses gliding strokes to knead the oil into your muscle and joints. The rubbing boosts circulation, relaxes the muscles, and loosens the joints. The therapists push down and swoop up your back nicely and rub your skin well, but Swedish massage therapists don't work the muscles as much as therapists who perform sports massage.

✔ **Sports massage:** This is the type of massage you want to search for. The main difference between Swedish and sports massage is that sports massage therapists use the palms of their hands to bear down on the sore muscles in the legs and back. They often use their fingers to apply pressure to areas of spasms. If you're just starting to get back in shape after years of inactivity, a sports massage should work out the kinks better than other types of massage.

✔ **Acupressure:** This is a Far East approach to bodywork. Acupressure is similar to acupuncture, but instead of sticking you with needles, the therapist uses his hands, elbows, knees, and feet to apply pressure to certain points of the body. If you've ever been elbowed on the basketball court, you know that you can figure on some discomfort while receiving acupressure. The Chinese believe that the best approach to relieving pressure to various organs and muscles is by stimulating the release of endorphins, the body's natural painkillers.

✔ **Reflexology:** Here's an interesting form of foot massage. In reflexology, you lie totally clothed on a padded table with your shoes and socks off. The reflexologist uses his thumbs and fingers to massage specific reflex zones on your feet, which proponents claim can successfully reduce low-back pain, chronic indigestion, and headaches.

✔ **Myofascial release:** This form of massage seeks to ease tension in your *fascia,* the soft connective tissues between muscles and bones. A physical therapist attempts to stretch this connective tissue with his fingers, palms, and elbows — the idea being that trauma, illness, or stress will cause your fascia to tighten up and pull bones and muscles out of place. The pressure should be light and not painful.

✔ **Rolfing:** Rolfing, which is another form of manipulating your fascia, had its heyday back when disco was king, but it's still alive and well today. Practitioners, who are called Rolfers (named after the person who invented Rolfing: biochemist Ida Rolf), employ deep, often painful pressure with fingers and elbows to reorganize your fascia to restore flexibility and relieve chronic pain.

My advice is to stick with a certified, traditional sports massage therapist who can work your muscles and joints without causing considerable pain. Massage helps increase blood and lymph flow, improves range of motion, helps repair fatigued or injured muscles, and hastens your recovery from overexertion. All of these benefits can aid you in your quest to be fit. A massage can also lift your spirits as endorphins are released into the bloodstream. If you can't afford a massage therapist on a regular basis, tell your partner that gift certificates make great presents!

Finding an Alternative to a Professional Massage

You probably already know this, but massage therapy is not cheap. Hour-long sessions can cost from $30 to $100, although some people opt for half-hour and 45-minute sessions to lower their cost.

If the choice is between making a car payment or scheduling a couple of massages, you can keep the Repo Man at bay by doing a self-massage or asking a family member to rub you down. These two approaches do have drawbacks, however:

- ✔ If you massage yourself, your body will not be totally relaxed. You can't reach your back, which often needs massage therapy the most in the middle-age years, and staying motivated to knead your muscles beyond a few minutes is often difficult.

- ✔ Having a spouse or family member give you a massage is like Amateur Night at the Comedy Club. Seriously, massage therapists undergo training for years, so you can't expect your spouse to give you a competent massage, but if he or she wants to try, it's going to be better than nothing. With some extra effort, he or she could do a fairly good job with your feet, calves, knees, ankles, wrists, forearms, upper arms, and shoulders.

And the news about self-massage isn't all bad, either. It can help you prevent muscle and tendon injuries by helping increase blood flow. You increase blood flow by kneading the area in a circular motion. Gradually increase pressure as you rub, but never to the point of pain. The idea is to loosen stiff, tight muscles with your fingers. Try it; you may like this form of massage.

Do I have to get naked?

Good question. No, great question. Disrobing in front of a stranger of either sex can cause a panic attack in even the most self-confident of people.

You are generally unclothed when receiving massage therapy, although I have received massages while wearing a one-piece or two-piece bathing suit. Massage therapists do not whip off the covering sheet to inspect your body. They often fold back a section of the white sheet to work on that area.

The last time I checked, massage therapists came in male and female forms, so if you would feel more comfortable with a same-sex therapist, you should have no problem finding one.

I have massaged myself frequently over the years. Just before the 1987 Wimbledon, my right elbow was so sore that I could not lift a coffee cup. I thought I would have to pull out for sure. My doctor, after injecting the area with a muscle relaxant, said that if I massaged my arm four times a day, I might be able to play. I moved those muscle fibers around at least four times a day in an attempt to bring more blood to the sore elbow. I'm glad I did; that year, I reached the finals of Wimbledon's Ladies Doubles, my best showing at tennis's biggest tournament.

But if you are going to massage yourself, ladies, be careful with those varicose veins, which often come to the surface after childbirth. Varicose veins should not be massaged because varicose veins are a form of *phlebitis,* or inflammation of the veins. Massage would just inflame the tender veins even more.

Part V

The Part of Tens

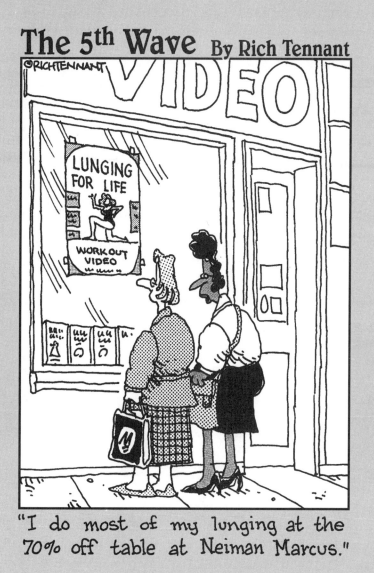

The 5th Wave By Rich Tennant

LUNGING FOR LIFE

WORK OUT VIDEO

"I do most of my lunging at the 70% off table at Neiman Marcus."

In this part . . .

The Dummies tradition of grouping key and fun information into easy-to-skim top-ten lists continues. You'll be inspired by ten great things that exercise can do for you and ten quotes featuring the wit and wisdom of people like Hippocrates, Sir Winston Churchill, and Will Rogers. This part also offers ten extreme and not-so-extreme sports that you should try someday and ten movies that you can rent to keep yourself motivated to exercise or play your favorite sport. You'll also want to check out an assessment of ten popular magazines about fitness and several Web sites you can visit for more fitness-related information.

Chapter 24

Ten Great Things That Exercise Can Do for You

In This Chapter

▶ Boosting your energy, correcting your coordination, and diminishing your anxiety

▶ Steeling your posture and putting an end to muscle deterioration

▶ Bettering your circulation, lowering your blood pressure, and showing off healthier skin

*W*hat if someone came up to you and asked, "How would you like to look younger, feel more confident — and be able to zip your favorite jeans without pliers?"

Naturally, you'd say, "Where do I sign up?" Well, when you resolve to do something about your fitness — and follow through on that promise to yourself — you and your body reap many benefits. Here are a few for your reading pleasure.

Gives You Energy

When you exercise, you increase the production of red blood cells, which in turn increases the amount of oxygen sent to your muscles. By increasing the amount of oxygen sent to your muscles, you increase your aerobic capacity and raise your fitness level. This improved fitness level enables you to go through your day with less expenditure of energy, leaving you with more energy at the end of the day — more gas in the tank. You may call upon your energy reserve when you need a second wind after the workday is over.

Prevents Muscle Deterioration

It's sad but true: As you age, the strength and size of your muscles decrease by 1 percent a year unless you embark on a steady, consistent exercise program. Lack of exercise causes your muscles to shrink, but exercising regularly helps your muscles rebuild themselves. To maintain muscle strength and size, combine aerobic exercise with strength training or lifting weights.

Helps Coordination

Not only do the strength and size of your muscles decrease with age, but your reflexes and coordination decline as well. You can help counter the decline in your muscle strength and coordination by exercising. Let me explain: In tennis, I practice making my forehand and backhand strokes the same way each time to create muscle memory. In the same way, when you repeat exercise movements through your athletic pursuits during your middle-age years, you keep your muscle memory; your reflexes and physical skills stay sharp.

Makes Your Skin Look Better

Worry about wrinkles? Wonder about crow's feet? Exercise increases blood flow to the skin; the increased blood flow provides nutrients your skin needs to stay thick. Thick skin wrinkles less than thin skin. If you are looking for a dramatic change that comes from facelifts or other cosmetic surgery, exercise may not replace the surgeon's scalpel, but exercise can give the body's covering a more healthful glow and possibly slow down the development of wrinkles.

Helps Prevent Osteoporosis

Women often experience weakening of their bones after menopause, and 20 percent of those suffering from osteoporosis — and stooped-over walks — are men. Walking can be a great antidote to osteoporosis. The results from a Tufts University study of older women show that walkers increase spinal bone size by 0.5 percent, while inactive women lose 7 percent of their bone mass. In addition, keep in mind that weight training, even for those in their sixties and up, can still strengthen bones through a buildup in bone density.

Prevents High Blood Pressure

When you reach middle age, you are more susceptible to developing high blood pressure because your heart's pumping capacity diminishes. Your heart is a muscle, and like all your muscles, its strength decreases as you age. Exercise plays an important role in keeping your heart in shape. In addition, when you exercise and lose weight, you decrease the amount of fat in your arteries, allowing the blood to flow more freely. When your arteries are open, your blood may flow more freely, making it easier for your heart to pump. Expanded arteries and a stronger heart mean lower blood pressure. If you can maintain your blood pressure at a low rate through exercise, you can avoid taking those strong medications designed to lower your blood pressure.

No Investing in a "Large" Wardrobe

Think of all the money you save by not shopping for new clothes because your size keeps fluctuating as you go on and off fad diets and trendy exercise programs. No more humiliating trips to Target to prowl the racks, searching for outfits to drape over your large, larger, or largest figure. One of the benefits of getting back into shape is losing weight and keeping it off, which means you can *reward* yourself with a new, smaller-sized, and more permanent wardrobe. In addition, the racks that hold the average sizes are plentiful and offer a wider variety of styles. (Not to mention that these clothes are more frequently on sale.) You'll look and feel like a winner in your new duds.

Makes You Fitter Than Young Couch Potatoes

Staying physically fit in your middle-age years may keep you as physically fit — or more physically fit — than persons years younger than your chronological age. In a Utah study, physically fit people in their mid-fifties were compared to inactive males in their mid-twenties. The older men had lower resting heart rates of 64 beats a minute, while the younger men had resting heart rates of 85 beats a minute. The older men also had higher oxygen intakes during exercise workouts and slower heart rates in the first minute after exercising. To add an additional insult, the middle-aged men weighed an average of 166 pounds, compared to 192 for the young loafers.

Helps You Lose Fat around Your Midsection

Yes, nearly all of us put on weight as we age. Many of us try to battle this weight gain by going on diets. A University of Washington study found that dieters must lose four times more weight than exercisers in order to lose the same amount of *central fat*. (Central fat is the fat that sits around your waist that may lead to heart disease.) The reason dieters must lose more weight in order to lose more fat is because exercisers lose weight by working hard to burn fat, and dieters lose weight by eating less.

Temporarily Reduces Anxiety

A good workout blows off steam! You may be aware of that fact, but did you realize that working out also allows you to shut off your brain and ignore other hassles in your life because you are concentrating on something else — your physical fitness? No wonder you feel refreshed after bone-tiring exercise.

Chapter 25

Ten Great Quotes about Exercise

. . . .

In This Chapter

▶ Wit and wisdom, from Hippocrates to Will Rogers

▶ Quotations that inspire you — and cause you to work your smiling muscles

▶ Messages that are both philosophical and practical

. . . .

I've always enjoyed pithy comments or interesting takes on life, exercise, and fitness. Here are a few pearls of wisdom from days past that are still applicable to our lives today (listed by their writer or speaker).

Benjamin Franklin

Printer, scientist, and writer, Benjamin Franklin became one of the great statesmen of the American Revolution and of the newborn nation. He was called the "wisest American" in his day.

"To lengthen thy life, lessen thy meals."

Hippocrates

Hippocrates, who lived from 460 to 370 B.C., is recognized as the father of medicine. After reading his quotation below, I would hazard a guess that this Greek scholar was the first person to say "use it or lose it."

"All parts of the body which have a function, if used in moderation and exercised in labors in which each is accustomed, become thereby healthy, well-developed, and age more slowly; but if unused and left idle they come liable to disease, defective in growth, and age quickly."

Mark Twain

Born Samuel Clemens, this nineteenth-century writer is best known for his seminal works *The Adventures of Tom Sawyer* and *The Adventures of Huckleberry Finn,* and for his wry sense of humor.

"I have never taken any exercise except sleeping and resting."

Thomas Jefferson

Author of the Declaration of Independence and third president of the United States, Thomas Jefferson was a scientist, architect, and a philosopher-statesman vitally interested in every phase of human activity.

"The sovereign invigorator of the body is exercise, and of all the exercises, walking is the best."

Mickey Mantle

Mickey Mantle, the larger-than-life New York Yankee who patrolled center field with grace and majesty in the 1950s and '60s, was also well known for his consumption of alcohol. One reason why Mickey drank was his suspicion that he would follow his father, grandfather, and two uncles to an early grave. He was 46 years old when he uttered the following quote, admittedly half in jest:

"If I knew I was going to live this long, I would have taken better care of myself."

Milton Berle

Comedian, entertainer, and *bon vivant*, "Uncle Miltie" was television's biggest star in its early days.

"It's rough to go through life with your contents looking as if they settled during shipping."

Unknown

I hope you enjoy this Italian proverb, which is *classico:*

> *"He who enjoys good health is rich, though he knows it not."*

John F. Kennedy

Before he was struck down by an assassin's bullet in Dallas, President John F. Kennedy was known for his "vim and vigah" as the 35th president of the United States. In 1960, at the age of 43, Kennedy was the youngest man ever elected president.

> *"We do not want in the United States a nation of spectators. We want a nation of participants in the vigorous life."*

Will Rogers

This cowboy philosopher and humorist from the 1920s and '30s was known for his salty comments on the political and social scenes.

> *"Even if you are on the right track, you'll get run over if you just sit there."*

Winston Churchill

British statesman, soldier, and author, Winston Churchill was prime minister of Great Britain during World War II. His stirring oratory during the darkest days of that war was crucial in rallying British resistance to the Nazi Germany threat.

> *"A fanatic is one who can't change his mind and won't change the subject."*

Chapter 26

Ten Extreme — and Not-So-Extreme — Sports to Try

In This Chapter

▶ Leaving your roller skates behind; some new ways to exercise

▶ Discovering some old ways to exercise that might be new to you

▶ Sneaking a little more fitness into your day

*R*eady to let your hair down? Don't have any hair to let down? Doesn't matter. It's time to spice up your fitness program with some new (or old, but different) sports and exercises — even thrills. Get out of the house, shake things up, cut loose, and don't stand still until you do something you've never done before.

I admit that some of these activities don't offer many fitness benefits, but they may act as confidence boosters that get your blood pumping. After trying a couple of these activities, you'll be thinking young and active.

Riding a Razor Scooter

Okay, it's the fad *du jour*. These shiny metallic scooters are equipped with two in-line–style wheels, a platform wide enough to fit an adult's foot, and a T-shaped handlebar. After a swift push, you speed along the sidewalk or street, feeling like a kid. You may continue to move quickly with a couple of foot pumps. (Some models of razor scooters fold up and fit inside a backpack.)

Bungee Jumping

Okay, it's not a sport, but bungee jumping sure looks like an activity that quickly raises your heart rate into the target zone. I stand in awe watching bungee jumpers leap off towers in Orlando, secured by only shoulder and seat harnesses. I see myself some day, standing on the railing of the bridge 1,000 feet over the valley, repeating over and over, "No risk . . . no risk." Or maybe I don't see myself. . . .

Cliff Diving

Now here's an extreme activity I *have* done. I was in Maui, and Miles Shanks, a tennis player who lived part-time in the Islands, showed me a great cliff-diving spot. Then Miles dared me to jump off a 50-foot cliff into the Pacific Ocean. "What's the matter?" he asked. "You chicken? My mom even jumped off." With friends egging me on, I succumbed to peer pressure. I dived off the cliff. About half-way down, I thought I had made the biggest mistake of my life. (That was nearly the same time that Miles muttered to bystanders, "I was just kidding. My mother never jumped off this cliff.") After hitting the water, I decided that cliff diving was one of the most exhilarating thrills I have experienced and obviously, I lived to tell about it.

Taking a Multisport Vacation

What a great way to scratch your *wanderlust* itch and enjoy a vacation that doesn't add extra double-digit pounds. Travel companies put together package tours in which you find yourself bicycling, hiking, kayaking, rafting, scuba diving, canoeing, sailing, cross-country skiing, or Alpine skiing in faraway locales. Instead of taking a bus tour through New England to see the fall colors, ask several couples to join you on an organized bike tour. The tour guide supplies the bikes, makes your reservations at country inns, and totes your bags to your next stop. The kinds of multisport vacations you can book range from South Africa hiking expeditions to Nepal treks. Check your Sunday newspaper travel sections or upscale travel magazines for ideas and leads. (Another source is Abercrombie & Kent, which can be found on the Internet at abercrombiekent.com.)

Playing on a Softball Team

Fast pitch or slow pitch, playing softball makes you feel like a kid again. And reliving your sandlot pastime may get you back in the gym. Your workouts may help to increase your stamina so you can last through the final inning. Although standing in the outfield, watching the grass grow as the pitcher takes his time between pitches, is not very tiring, being part of this sport may rekindle your appreciation for spending an afternoon in the fresh air with your buddies. Play ball!

Riding a Street Luge

I know, it sounds ridiculous — riding on your back on a glorified skateboard down a steep street. But some folks get their kicks out of this sport. For me, the conditions and the gear must be perfect: a $2,000 professional leather "Power Ranger" suit; a luge with an aluminum chassis, custom seat, foot pegs, hand holds, lean-activated steering, and custom urethane wheels; a DOT-approved full-face helmet; leather gloves; and high-top, rubber-soled athletic shoes. Oh, and I also want a national ESPN audience watching me do the stupidest stunt I ever attempt.

Bobsledding

You may risk life and limb on the world's scariest bobsledding run at St. Moritz' Cresta Run, *and* the ride costs you an arm and a leg — 200 Swiss francs (or around $120) — for a one-minute replay of what the Jamaican bobsled team felt the first time they careened down the icy track. Don't worry, the Swiss provide the driver and the brakeman. You sit in the number 2 or 3 slot as the bobsled speeds down the icy track.

Mountain Biking Downhill-Style

Okay, here's the last downhill sport. Did you know that you can ride a mountain bike down a ski run? Every summer, more and more ski areas such as Vail and Copper Mountain in Colorado and Mammoth Mountain in California let mountain bikers ride up the gondolas with their bikes; then they ride down the ski trails. Mammoth has been the site for the skiing U.S. Nationals and includes a run appropriately called the "Kamikaze." You don't *have* to go downhill when mountain biking at a ski resort. Going up, down, and around the mountain could be a lung-expanding journey.

Surfing

If this old dog ever learns a new trick, I hope it's learning how to surf. Although I grew up in St. Petersburg and close to the beach, many people don't realize that the sheltered Gulf of Mexico doesn't produce large waves. I tried surfing a couple of times in Hawaii without success, but I'd like to give it another try someday on foam-like trainer boards. Don't forget that surfing is good exercise because you work your arms paddling the board out to the waves after each ride.

White-Water Rafting

I'm not talking about a serene raft trip along an oversized brook, but a full-bore, ride-'em-cowboy thrill ride. White-water rafting in Category III or IV rapids in a turbulent mountain stream is very exciting. The idea of those rafts bobbing up and down in a foamy cascade of water seems like too much fun to pass up! My only white-water–rafting experience happened on the Snake River outside Jackson Hole, Wyoming. I had a blast and worked my arms all afternoon long.

Paintball

You may think of paintball as a silly war-game exercise that appeals only to a certain segment of society (namely, testosterone-charged boys). But just once, I think I would like to try this game. I believe I would enjoy taking to the hills with my trusty paintball gun, carrying plenty of ammo, and trying to get the enemy before he/she gets me. With a straight face, I assure you that paintball offers fitness benefits. Running around backcountry terrain, weighted down by camouflage gear, gives you a serious workout.

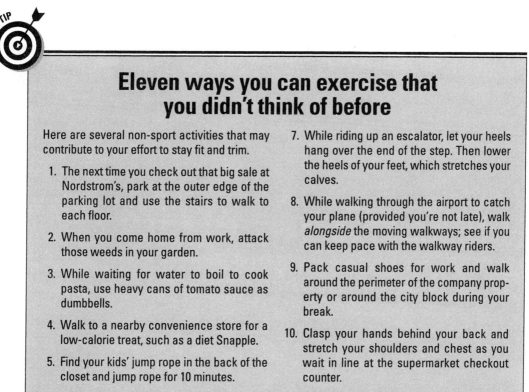

Eleven ways you can exercise that you didn't think of before

Here are several non-sport activities that may contribute to your effort to stay fit and trim.

1. The next time you check out that big sale at Nordstrom's, park at the outer edge of the parking lot and use the stairs to walk to each floor.

2. When you come home from work, attack those weeds in your garden.

3. While waiting for water to boil to cook pasta, use heavy cans of tomato sauce as dumbbells.

4. Walk to a nearby convenience store for a low-calorie treat, such as a diet Snapple.

5. Find your kids' jump rope in the back of the closet and jump rope for 10 minutes.

6. Take stairs two at a time, especially at work.

7. While riding up an escalator, let your heels hang over the end of the step. Then lower the heels of your feet, which stretches your calves.

8. While walking through the airport to catch your plane (provided you're not late), walk *alongside* the moving walkways; see if you can keep pace with the walkway riders.

9. Pack casual shoes for work and walk around the perimeter of the company property or around the city block during your break.

10. Clasp your hands behind your back and stretch your shoulders and chest as you wait in line at the supermarket checkout counter.

11. While driving home with your spouse some weekend day, ask him or her to drop you off a mile from home. Then walk!

Chapter 27

Ten Popular Magazines — and Some Great Web Sites, Too

In This Chapter

▶ Perusing your local newsstand or bookstore for magazines devoted to the pursuit of good health

▶ Clicking a mouse: Narrowing down the Internet options on health topics

*I*f you've developed a new appetite for exercise, you may be hungry for more fitness-related information. Health-and-fitness magazines are a great place to read up on exercise routines, new ways to work out, and what to eat and what to avoid in your diet. I like thumbing through a fitness magazine while I use my treadmill because my head is into this info during this time. Another fantastic source — and one getting better every day — is the Information Superhighway, where 1,782,645 pages on fitness are waiting for you on the Internet.

The Ink-on-Paper Versions: Fitness Magazines

Fitness magazines provide readers with fact-filled features, illuminating how-to articles, short takes, and tons of advertisements (some of which are interesting). After perusing the landscape, I now present you with the skinny on fitness magazines that appeal to those of us 40 and up. (By the way, *all* fitness magazines, even if they are targeted at young pups under 40, contain beneficial information to middle-aged readers.) The following periodicals are not ranked in any particular order, however.

Health

Target audience: Predominantly women, ages 30 to 55.

Editorial focus: Articles touch on a wide range of health-related topics such as fitness, dieting, skin care, recipes, and relationships.

My take: An excellent magazine that covers the topic of all-around fitness with a good mix of short and long articles.

Prevention

Target audience: Both sexes, 40 to 65 years of age.

Editorial focus: Follows a natural approach to health with many articles keying on herbs, vitamins, and proper nutrition.

My take: *Prevention* comes in the same size packaging as *Reader's Digest*, so it's easy to carry around. Besides being lightweight, *Prevention* has pleasing graphics and lively writing. *Prevention* will inspire you to watch what you eat and encourage you to look your best. If I had to criticize *Prevention*, it would be that the models look *too* good.

New Choices

Target audience: Both sexes, ages 50 to 60.

Editorial focus: Foods that fight disease, nutritious recipes, planning vacation cruises, and paying off medical bills are among this magazine's topics.

My take: *New Choices*, which is published by the *Reader's Digest* franchise, offers itself as a magazine for "living even better after age 50." *Prevention* serves the same audience better, however.

Walking

Target audience: Women, ages 30 to 55.

Editorial focus: A lot more than walking. In addition, any time celebrities may be connected to the topic of walking, you read about it. The magazine is filled with fitness tips, dieting articles, and suggested escapes to foreign locales where the walking is fun.

My take: This magazine took me by surprise. I didn't expect a magazine simply titled *Walking* to be this interesting.

Men's Health

Target audience: Sex-eager men, ages 20 to 35.

Editorial focus: Explains how men can develop killer abs and perform well in bed.

My take: Not favorable for this testosterone-juiced fitness title.

Men's Journal

Target audience: Men, ages 30 to 50.

Editorial focus: This magazine covers the three F's: fashion, fitness, and food. These main features are given plenty of editorial room, plus you may look at full-page photos in this *Rolling Stone*–sized periodical.

My take: I welcome this grown-up version of *Men's Health*.

Men's Fitness

Target audience: Serious fitness fanatics of the male persuasion, ages 25 to 45.

Editorial focus: Workouts, workouts, and more workouts — plenty of editorial space is devoted to equipment for the gear-head crowd.

My take: If you join a heavy-duty fitness emporium like Gold's Gym after reading this book, subscribe to this magazine.

Ageless

Target audience: Both sexes, ages 45 to 65.

Editorial focus: Articles discuss the style and wisdom of today's mature adults — features on skin care, fashion, and making the most of your remaining years.

My take: An excellent periodical for those with maybe a touch of gray in their hair.

Fitness

Target audience: Active women, ages 25 to 45.

Editorial focus: Features focus on women who want to look good and feel good. Articles on beauty, fashion, exercise, diet, and sports help women maintain a healthy and well-rounded lifestyle.

My take: Another keeper. *Fitness* is a well-rounded periodical in tremendous tip-top shape.

Life Extension

Target audience: Men and women, ages 50 and up.

Editorial focus: Articles center on how to live longer and extend your life span, featuring topics about dealing with health issues and the latest medical findings on slowing and reversing aging.

My take: The quasi-spiritual tones underlying the articles is off-putting, and the writers' voices seem desperate, focusing on doing *anything* to live longer instead of making the most of the present. Skip this one.

The World Wide Web of Fitness

Pinpointing the best fitness-related Web sites is like pinpointing the best place to lay a towel on a beach. The Web offers just too many possibilities. Obviously, playing around with your favorite search engine by typing in "fitness" or "fitness over 40" is a way to engage the incredible resources of the Internet. I don't want to send you away empty-handed, however, so here are a few Web sites worth checking out:

✔ fitnesslink.com is a comprehensive Web site that posts a new health-related story each day. The content covers the fitness waterfront; you can find articles on everything from aerobics to yoga on this site. The graphics are excellent.

✔ efit.com is another mega-site with a wide-ranging list of articles; channels to various sporting interests (walking, tennis, and so forth); healthy living tools (body mass index and other fitness calculators); and healthy living portals that lead you to hundreds of other fitness-related sites.

✔ epinions.com is a good place to find out what others just like *you* think about fitness club chains (Bally, L.A. Fitness), strength-training equipment, home equipment, and fitness magazines. You may find the reading to be spicy and highly entertaining.

✔ prevention.com is provided by the same company that produces *Prevention* magazine, and its Web site is certainly worth checking out. (The content mirrors that in the magazine; see earlier comments.)

Chapter 28

Ten Great Motivating Movies

In This Chapter

▶ Soaking up some inspiration from the screen

▶ Laughing — or crying — with notable sports-world characters

*N*eed an emotional lift to inspire you to greater heights in your fitness or sports regimen? Do you like watching movies in which sports play a prominent role? Then walk, don't run, to your nearest video store and rent one of the following films that will motivate you to stay with the program — and tug at your heart strings or deliver loads of laughs. These movies might energize you to keep working out in the face of impossible odds — a hectic work schedule, a demanding home front, or years of inactivity. Happy endings don't happen just in Hollywood.

Chariots of Fire

Exhibitions of good sportsmanship are rare these days, which is why this stirring story of Eric Lidell and the British track team during the 1924 Olympics tops my list. Winner of the Oscar for Best Picture, this 1981 film highlights such commendable qualities as commitment, perseverance, and fraternity. You'll also feel like going for a long run the next time you visit a wide, sandy beach.

Field of Dreams

In the middle of an Iowa cornfield, Ray Kinsella hears a voice telling him, "If you build it, he will come," which leads the viewer down a path full of mystery, magic, and baseball. When Ray (played by Kevin Costner) finally gets to play catch with his dad, I well up.

Rocky

"Yo, Adrian!" I'm talking about the original *Rocky* movie — the rags-to-riches story of a Philly club fighter who rises from obscurity to get a shot at the world boxing championship. (Forget those lousy sequels — *Rocky II, III, IV, V, ad nauseum*.) *Rocky* tells a timeless story about how hard work and unyielding effort will help you reach your goals. If Bill Conti's title song, "Gonna Fly Now," doesn't pump you up, nothing will.

White Men Can't Jump

Woody Harrelson plays a white con artist who hustles basketball games with black players who smugly believe that white men can't jump — which makes them patsies on the court. When Wesley Snipes, an African American, agrees to become Woody's "agent" in these gambling basketball games, the plot gets interesting. Watching this movie really makes you want to hit the courts on a warm, sunny day for a pickup game of hoops.

Rudy

"Ru-dee! Ru-dee! Ru-dee!" Undersized, undertalented, and underfunded Daniel "Rudy" Ruettiger Jr. wants to play football at Notre Dame in the worst way in this touching film about how persistence, determination, and character can enable anyone to overcome great odds. Rudy ignores the limits that others (including his family) place on him and puts everything he has into chasing his dream — suiting up in a Fighting Irish football uniform. It's amazing how far his determination takes him, which is an apt reminder that you can succeed against tremendous odds as well.

Hoosiers

Gene Hackman plays a basketball coach who winds up coaching a small town high school basketball team in Indiana. He gets off to a bad start, and the locals dislike him; then he works his coaching magic, and his starting five become the Little Team That Could in this true story from the 1950s. Sure, the outcome is predictable, but you appreciate the journey that these Hoosier basketball players take on their route to playing for the state title.

Players

One of the few sports films centered on the tennis world, *Players* is a double-fault on break point. This 1979 film stars the late Dean Paul Martin (the son of late entertainer Dean Martin and a pretty fair tennis player) and Ali McGraw in a ludicrous romance (she being in her early forties, he being in his mid-twenties). The cameos of John McEnroe, Ilie Nastase, Pancho Gonzalez, and Guillermo Vilas are enjoyable to watch, but only Hollywood could script a final on Wimbledon's grass Centre Court between Vilas, a clay-courter, and the unseeded Dean Paul Martin. Despite the film's shortcomings, tennis enthusiasts will enjoy the athleticism and personalities of the real-life players.

Brian's Song

Look for this classic TV movie from 1971 in video stores or when it's reprised on cable TV. Gale Sayers (played by Billy Dee Williams) and Brian Piccolo (played by James Caan) are first seen as rookies trying to make the Chicago Bears football team. Sayers doesn't have to work too hard — he becomes a Hall of Fame runner — but Piccolo works extra hard just to be second best. The two players are selected to be the first interracial roommates back in the 1960s, and they become quite a team. Brian helps Gale rehabilitate a knee injury, and Gale supports Brian during a bout with cancer, which eventually claims Brian's life in a tear-jerker ending.

Endless Summer

It's hard to believe that this original "stoke" film was made way back in 1964 by Bruce Brown. Simply put, this classic surf movie is a photo journal of two sunburnt guys on a globe-trotting journey to find the perfect wave. Great photography, funny story line, and an interesting take on the surfing culture of the sixties.

Follow the Sun

Never heard of this movie? I hadn't either, but my husband, Mark, says this biographical film about golfing legend Ben Hogan can raise the spirits of anyone who's down in the dumps. "Bantam Ben," as he was called, was one of the world's best golfers until a devastating automobile accident nearly claimed his life in 1949. The movie tells the story of his comeback against tremendous odds. Starring Glenn Ford as Ben Hogan, this movie can be found at well-stocked video stores, or it is sometimes featured on the Golf Channel.

Index

Notes

Notes

Notes

Notes

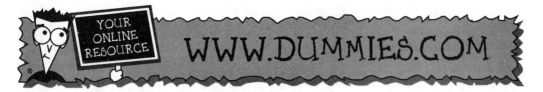

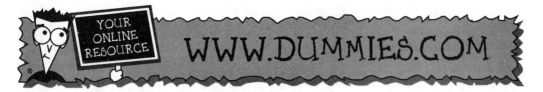

Discover Dummies Online!

The Dummies Web Site is your fun and friendly online resource for the latest information about *For Dummies®* books and your favorite topics. The Web site is the place to communicate with us, exchange ideas with other *For Dummies* readers, chat with authors, and have fun!

Ten Fun and Useful Things You Can Do at www.dummies.com

1. Win free *For Dummies* books and more!

2. Register your book and be entered in a prize drawing.

3. Meet your favorite authors through the IDG Books Worldwide Author Chat Series.

4. Exchange helpful information with other *For Dummies* readers.

5. Discover other great *For Dummies* books you must have!

6. Purchase Dummieswear® exclusively from our Web site.

7. Buy *For Dummies* books online.

8. Talk to us. Make comments, ask questions, get answers!

9. Download free software.

10. Find additional useful resources from authors.

Link directly to these ten fun and useful things at **http://www.dummies.com/10useful**

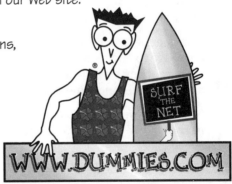

For other technology titles from IDG Books Worldwide, go to www.idgbooks.com

Not on the Web yet? It's easy to get started with *Dummies 101®: The Internet For Windows® 98* or *The Internet For Dummies®* at local retailers everywhere.

Find other *For Dummies* books on these topics:

Business • Career • Databases • Food & Beverage • Games • Gardening • Graphics • Hardware
Health & Fitness • Internet and the World Wide Web • Networking • Office Suites
Operating Systems • Personal Finance • Pets • Programming • Recreation • Sports
Spreadsheets • Teacher Resources • Test Prep • Word Processing

IDG BOOKS WORLDWIDE BOOK REGISTRATION

Register This Book and Win!

We want to hear from you!

Visit **http://my2cents.dummies.com** to register this book and tell us how you liked it!

✔ Get entered in our monthly prize giveaway.

✔ Give us feedback about this book — tell us what you like best, what you like least, or maybe what you'd like to ask the author and us to change!

✔ Let us know any other *For Dummies*® topics that interest you.

Your feedback helps us determine what books to publish, tells us what coverage to add as we revise our books, and lets us know whether we're meeting your needs as a *For Dummies* reader. You're our most valuable resource, and what you have to say is important to us!

Not on the Web yet? It's easy to get started with *Dummies 101*®*: The Internet For Windows*® *98* or *The Internet For Dummies*® at local retailers everywhere.

Or let us know what you think by sending us a letter at the following address:

For Dummies Book Registration
Dummies Press
10475 Crosspoint Blvd.
Indianapolis, IN 46256

™

...FOR DUMMIES

BESTSELLING BOOK SERIES